Reactions to Psychotropic Medication

Reactions to Psychotropic Medication

Frank L. Tornatore, Pharm.D.
Assistant Professor of Clinical Pharmacy
University of Southern California School of Pharmacy
Los Angeles, California

John J. Sramek, Pharm.D.
Drug Information Specialist
Department of Pharmaceutical Services
and Assistant Director
Clinical Research Unit
Metropolitan State Hospital
Norwalk, California

Bette L. Okeya, Pharm.D.
Clinical Pharmacist
Department of Pharmaceutical Services
UCLA Medical Center
and Neuropsychiatric Institute
Los Angeles, California

and

Edmond H. Pi, M.D.
Associate Professor
Department of Psychiatry
University of Southern California School of Medicine
Los Angeles, California

PLENUM MEDICAL BOOK COMPANY
NEW YORK AND LONDON

Library of Congress Cataloging in Publication Data

Reactions to psychotropic medication.

Bibliography: p.
Includes index.
1. Psychotropic drugs—Side effects. 2. Psychotropic drugs—Toxicology. I.
Tornatore, Frank L. [DNLM: 1. Psychopharmacology. 2. Psychotropic Drugs—
adverse effects. QV 77 R282]
RM315.R43 1987   615'.788   87-30056
ISBN-13: 978-1-4684-5414-7   e-ISBN-13: 978-1-4684-5412-3
DOI: 10.1007/978-1-4684-5412-3

© 1987 Plenum Publishing Corporation
Softcover reprint of the hardcover 1st edition 1987
233 Spring Street, New York, N.Y. 10013

Plenum Medical Book Company is an imprint of
Plenum Publishing Corporation

Preface

After thousands of clinical trials, the efficacy of psychotropic drugs in the treatment of psychiatric disorders has become well established. However, the very success of these drugs has meant that many patients with chronic illnesses will receive them for a significant part of their lifetime. Side effects and other adverse reactions are an unfortunate but unavoidable component of successful pharmacotherapy. Indeed, the main emphasis in new drug development is often on the search for compounds that have fewer side effects, although no one has as yet found an effective drug without them. Therefore, it is important for clinicians to be aware of side effect reaction profiles, because they are often a major determining factor in the choice of therapy.

After more than three decades of major breakthroughs in the development of psychotropic drugs, reactions to these medications are still frequently reported in the current literature, and information about well-known reactions is constantly refined. This book is an attempt to systematically collect and organize this large body of data and present it in an easy-to-use form. All chapters follow the same reaction-oriented logic, and each important reaction is discussed using the same consistent subdivisions. The more clinically important reactions appear in the body of each chapter; the more unusual or rarely reported reactions are briefly characterized in the miscellaneous section at the end of each chapter.

This manual is meant to supplement other sources of information in psychopharmacology, and we hope that it will serve as the impetus for further readings in this field. The

authors will be pleased if clinicians find this work to be a
handy reference in daily practice as an aid to improving
patient care.

John J. Sramek, Pharm.D.
Frank L. Tornatore, Pharm.D.

Contents

Chapter 2
Reactions to Antidepressants: Tricyclic and
Tetracyclic

Reactions to Psychotropic Medication

1

Reactions to Antipsychotics

AUTONOMIC EFFECTS

Anticholinergic Effects

Anticholinergic Properties of Some Common Neuroleptics	
High Anticholinergic Properties	
Clozaril (clozapine) Mellaril (thioridazine) Serentil (mesoridazine)	Thorazine (chlorpromazine) Stelazine (trifluoperazine)
Low Anticholinergic Properties	
Navane (thiothixene) Moban (molindone) Loxapine (loxitane)	Prolixin (fluphenazine) Haldol (haloperidol)

Dry Mouth

Presentation and Clinical Significance. There is decreased saliva secretion. The patient frequently complains of thirst or dry mouth.

Dry mouth is very common; tolerance may develop. Dry mouth may dispose the patient to develop monilial infection

---

The terms *antipsychotic* and *neuroleptic* are used interchangeably in this handbook.

(which appears as a creamy white curdlike patch); this
infection has been most often reported with thioridazine.

Recommendations. Sugarless gum or candy, frequent
mouth-rinsing or sips of water, and ice chips may help
relieve dry mouth. If monilial infection occurs, start anti-
fungal therapy with nystatin oral suspension.

Constipation

Presentation and Mechanism. Decreased gastrointestinal
motility (intestinal tone and peristalsis) and decreased secretions. Constipation can be accompanied by pain, abdominal
distention, rigidity, and vomiting.

Recommendations. Mild cases of constipation can be
treated with diet, adequate fluids, and exercise. More severe
cases of constipation can be treated with various choices of
laxatives (stool softener, bulk forming, saline types, or
stimulants). Laxatives should be used in the lowest effective
dose and as infrequently as possible, particularly the stimulant (cathartic) types. Many clinicians recommend a stool
softener such as DOSS (Docusate Sodium) with 8 oz of
water.

Paralytic Ileus

Presentation. Usual symptoms include constipation, abdominal distention, and discomfort.

Clinical Significance. If left untreated, paralytic ileus
may result in death. In 6 of 13 cases reported (see Bluhm
and Koller, 1981), drug doses were higher than what is
commonly recommended for maintenance therapy. The higher
doses given were of either an antipsychotic or an anticholinergic or a combination of both, which resulted in the
development of paralytic ileus (of the reported cases, 11 of

13 received an aliphatic or piperidine phenothiazine; 12 of 13 received a second drug high in anticholinergic properties, primarily an antiparkinson agent or, less often, a tricyclic antidepressant). Severe cases may require treatment in an acute medical setting.

Recommendations. Discontinue or lower the dose of the offending agent, if risk outweighs benefit. Early detection of symptoms can be treated symptomatically with success, but if the dosage of the offending agent is not reduced, the condition may recur.

If treatment is necessary:

1. Correct fluid and electrolyte balance.
2. Alleviate vomiting and distention of the abdomen by intubation of the gut and relief of pressure.
3. Restore bowel continuity and function.

Blurred Vision

Presentation. Patient complains of blurred vision, especially when reading.

Mechanism. Blurred vision results from paralyzed (relaxed) ciliary muscle, which dilates the pupil and flattens the lens to accommodate for distant vision but not for near vision (loss of accommodation for near vision).

Clinical Significance. Dilation of the pupil will precipitate closure of the anterior chamber angle, which may exacerbate an existing narrow-angle glaucoma. Symptoms may include recurrent episodes of blurred vision with pain in or around the eye or rainbow-colored rings seen around lights at night. If existing glaucoma is being treated, there is no cause to worry. Open-angle glaucoma is due to excessive resistance in outflow channels (mainly within the trabecular meshwork) and is not affected by dilation of the pupil. Tolerance to the blurred vision may develop with time.

Recommendations.
1. Decrease the dose of the offending agent.
2. Switch to another agent with lower anticholinergic properties.

Urinary Retention

Presentation. Overdistention of the bladder, discomfort, pain, and possibly bladder infection. Older male patients with benign prostatic hypertrophy are particularly prone to develop urinary retention.

Recommendations.
1. Discontinue the offending agent or reduce the dosage.
2. Consider a trial of bethanechol, 10–25 mg TID.

Tachycardia (Ventricular)

Presentation. Heart beat races, palpitation.

Clinical Significance. The significance of ventricular tachycardia has not been established. Some tolerance to this effect does develop. Tachycardia may prove problematic in patients with an underlying cardiac disturbance or in the elderly.

Suggested Readings

Bluhm R. E., Koller W. C.: Anticholinergic abuse—when to suspect it, what to do about it. *Drug Ther* 1981:150–155, 1981.

Heiser J. F., Gilli J. C.: The reversal of anticholinergic drug induced delirium and coma with physostigmine. *Am J Psychiatry* 127:1050–1054, 1971.

Johnson A. L., Hollister L. E., Berger P. A.: The anticholinergic intoxication syndrome: Diagnosis and treatment. *J Clin Psychiatry* 42(8):313–317, 1981.

Katz T. M.: Intraocular pressure decrease in normal volunteers following timolol ophthalmic solution. *Invest Ophthalmol* 15:489, 1976.

Lang A. W., Moore R. A.: Acute toxic psychosis concurrent with phenothiazine therapy. *Am J Psychiatry* 128:95–99, 1971.

Marmion V. J.: Trends in ocular therapeutics. *Practitioner* 1980:609–630, 1980.
Reid W. H., Rakes S.: Intraocular pressure in patients receiving psychotropic medication. *Psychosomatics* 24:665–667, 1983.

Temperature Regulation

Presentation

In very hot weather (usually heat waves of 100°F or more), a patient whose temperature-regulating mechanisms are impaired by neuroleptics may present with high temperature (42°C rectal), hot dry skin, altered level of consciousness, seizures, altered respirations, and circulatory collapse. This would be a case of drug-induced hyperpyrexia, but one must also keep in mind that shivering and freezing could be seen in very cold temperatures.

Incidence

The incidence is not well known, but is a function of the drugs ingested, the extremes of environmental temperature (e.g., very hot or very cold), plus individual vulnerability factors (see Clinical Significance) and individual predisposition.

Mechanism

Neuroleptics interfere with the temperature-regulating function of the hypothalamus and can also interfere peripherally with the sweating mechanism. The result is poikilothermy, in which temperature regulation is controlled primarily by environmental influence.

Clinical Significance

Hyperpyrexia and hypothermia are both potentially life-threatening conditions. Hyperpyrexia can lead to heat stroke with massive damage to the circulatory system and the central nervous system (CNS). Therefore, it is particularly important to pay attention to vulnerability factors. In addition to temperature extremes, patients taking neuroleptic medication may also be at risk for hyperpyrexia if they are overweight, physically active to the point of fatigue, using alcohol, or also taking high doses of antiparkinson agents, which add to the already inherent anticholinergic effects of certain neuroleptics. Older patients and those with organic brain syndromes will also be more vulnerable.

Recommendations

The most important aspect is prevention which is accomplished by paying attention to risk factors (see Incidence and Clinical Significance), especially in vulnerable patients during periods of extreme ambient temperatures. Prevention is particularly important because of the high mortality associated with hyper- and hypothermic states. If a patient develops hyperpyrexia, the primary efforts should be supportive, body temperature must be lowered (ice baths), lost fluids must be replaced, and the body's acid–base balance must be corrected. In extreme cases, anticoagulants are administered to prevent intravascular coagulation and diazepam or other antiepileptics are given to prevent seizures.

Suggested Readings

Mann S. C., Boger W. P.: Psychotropic drugs, summer heat and humidity, and hyperpyrexia: A danger restated. *Am J Psychiatry* 135:1097–1100, 1978.

Noto T. N., Hashimoto H., Sugae S., *et al.*: Hypothermia caused by antipsychotic drugs in a schizophrenic patient. *J Clin Psychiatry* 48:77–78, 1987.

Penovich P.: Drug-induced hyperpyrexia and heat stroke. *Drug Ther* 1976:101–102, August 1976.

CARDIOVASCULAR EFFECTS

Electrocardiographic Effects

Presentation

The types of electrocardiographic (ECG) changes seen are those of conduction defects. You may see blunted, notched, broadened, inverted T waves; a depressed ST segment; an increased QT interval; or appearance of U waves. The occurrence of serious arrhythmias is rare, but can be life-threatening (e.g., Torsade de Pointes reported with thioridazine).

Incidence

ECG changes are most frequently reported with piperidine phenothiazines, then aliphatic phenothiazines, then piperazine phenothiazines. No incidence is reported for other neuroleptics, but one may assume it is similar to that of the piperazine phenothiazines.

Gender and duration of therapy do not influence the incidence of ECG changes seen. Elderly patients show more changes, which may be attributed to the higher probability of a compromised cardiac status.

Mechanism

The mechanism is as yet unknown, but there are postulated causes:

1. A direct myocardial depressant effect, rather than an autonomic or central effect.
2. A shift of potassium intracellularly, thereby modifying repolarization and decreasing intracellular sodium.
3. Chelation of magnesium and calcium, which may disrupt cardiac enzymatic action.
4. Alteration of catecholamine concentrations (decreased

reuptake in cardiac tissue and increased circulating level).
5. Acid mucopolysaccharide lesions in arterioles and myocardial tissue, causing ischemia and necrosis.

Clinical Significance

Several factors may predispose a patient to the cardiac effects of antipsychotics:

1. Exercise: Strenuous exercise for a patient on moderate to high doses may be hazardous.
2. Hypokalemia: Arrhythmias are associated with low potassium (<3.0 meq/liter) in nonmedicated patients. There is a rare occurrence of phenothiazine-induced arrhythmias with normal potassium levels.
3. High doses: They increase the risk of cardiac complications.
4. Preexisting cardiac disease.
5. Other drugs that cause ECG changes, e.g., tricyclic antidepressants when given concomitantly with neuroleptics.

Thioridazine is particularly implicated in causing ECG changes, specifically T-wave changes. These changes have been noted at low doses and invariably at large doses (2–3 times greater than the maximum allowed by the FDA). T-wave changes are often seen in normal, healthy, physically active patients. Thioridazine-induced T waves seen in patients with normal cardiac status have been described as "benign" (with no evidence of organic heart disease). A simple test has been recommended to determine whether the wave change is "benign" or one of organic nature. A "benign" T-wave change will revert to normal with either of the following: (1) rapid-acting nitrate (isosorbide dinitrate, 10 mg sublingual), shortly after one is taken; or (2) a 10-g mixture of potassium salts (5 g potassium citrate and 5 g potassium acetate), within 1 hr. (This test is not recommended for patients with renal insufficiency, recent myocardial infarction, or acute myocarditis.)

It has also been suggested that thioridazine T-wave

changes are "quinidinelike," but this point is not yet clear. Unlike quinidine-induced changes, thioridazine T-wave changes are reversible with administration of nitrate or potassium, do not depress ventricular function, and do not widen the QRS interval.

"Benign" T-wave changes (in patients with normal cardiac status) will disappear after the drug is discontinued.

Recommendations

1. Take a base-line and follow-up ECGs on patients with increased risk factors.
2. Avoid the use of strongly anticholinergic phenothiazines, especially in the elderly or those with a compromised cardiac status.
3. Consider a butyrophenone (haloperidol) or other low-potency antipsychotic.

Suggested Readings

Alexander C. S., Nino A.: Cardiovascular complications in young patients taking psychotropic drugs. *Am Heart J* 78:757–769, 1969.

Alvarez-Mena S. C., Frank M. J.: Phenothiazine induced T wave abnormalities. *J Am Med Assoc* 224:1730–1733, 1973.

Fowler N. O. *et al.:* Electrocardiographic changes and cardiac arrhythmias in patients receiving psychotropic drugs. *Am J Cardiol* 37:223–230, 1976.

Patterson J. H., Pittman A. W., Willis P. W.: Drug induced changes in the electrocardiogram. *US Pharm* 8:46–52, 1983.

Risch S. C., Groom G. P., Janowsky D. S.: The effects of psychotropic drugs on the cardiovascular system. *J Clin Psychiatry* 43(5)(Sect 2):16–26, 1982.

Wilson W. H., Weilser S. J.: Case report of phenothiazine induced Torsade de Pointes. *Am J Psychiatry* 141:1265–1266, 1984.

Yoon M. S. *et al.:* Effects of thioridazine on ventricular electrophysiological properties. *Am J Cardiol* 43:1155–1158, 1979.

Postural Hypotension

Presentation

Blood pressure alterations are most prominent with aliphatic or piperidine phenothiazines. Generally, the risk of hypotension is increased with parenteral administration or very large dose changes. The geriatric population often presents with postural hypotension in the unmedicated state; therefore, a cautious approach is required when initiating medication in this group of patients. The most common predisposing factors to develop hypotension are age and cardiovascular disorders.

Incidence

One study reported an incidence of 41% within the first 72 hr of therapy, with only 18% of the patients symptomatic with mild complaints (i.e., dizziness) (see Jefferson, 1974).

Mechanism

These drugs may act at different levels of the blood pressure regulatory system (central and peripheral):

1. Centrally, to depress the vasomotor regulatory systems.
2. Peripherally, to depress cardiovascular reflexes.
3. Peripherally, to block α-adrenergic receptors, which contribute to maintenance of vasomotor tone. Blockade results in loss of vasoconstricting ability necessary to prevent venous pooling during postural changes.

Recommendations

1. With the systolic pressure below 90 mm Hg, it is advisable to withhold or reduce the dosage of neuroleptic. You may place the patient in the shock position (legs elevated).
2. Prevention of hypotensive episodes:
   a. Increase the dose gradually when initiating antipsychotic therapy.
   b. Warn the patient about the possibility that hypotension will occur and instruct the patient to stand slowly when rising from a reclining position to

allow time for circulatory compensation to occur (especially with the aliphatic and piperidine phenothiazines).
  c. Use elastic stockings in elderly patients to prevent pooling of blood in the extremities.
3. Drug treatment is not necessary unless shock develops:
  a. Epinephrine—the unopposed β-agonist activity can lead to further decrease in blood pressure; therefore, the following agents are preferred:
  b. Norepinephrine (Levarterenol, Levophen)—α, β
  c. Phenylephrine (Isophrin, Neo-Synephrine):
      i. Mild to moderate hypotension: 2–5 mg IM/SC. Initial dose should not exceed 5 mg.
      ii. Severe hypotension: 0.1–0.5 mg IV push, not to be repeated more than every 10–15 min. May also be given as a 10-mg infusion in 500 ml D5W or NS. Start the infusion at 100–180 drops/min, with a maintenance rate of 40–60 drops/min when the blood pressure is stabilized.
  d. Metaraminol (Aramine):
      i. Mild to moderate hypotension: 2–10 mg IM/SC.
      ii. Severe hypotension: 0.5–5 mg IV push followed by an infusion of 15–100 mg in 500 ml D5W.

Suggested Readings

Jefferson J.: Hypotension from drugs. *Dis Nerv Syst* 1974:66–71, 1974.
Koral B., Lang W. J., et al.: Effect of chronic chlorpromazine administration on systemic arterial pressure in schizophrenic patient—Relationship of body position to blood pressure. *Clin Pharmacol Ther* 1965:587–591, 1965.
Risch S. C., Groom G. P., Janowsky D. S.: Interfaces of psychopharmacology and cardiology—Part II. *J Clin Psychiatry* 42(2):47–57, 1981.
Rosati D.: Hypotensive side effects of phenothiazines and their management. *Dis Nerv Syst* 1964:366–369, 1964.

Witton K.: Orthostatic hypotension secondary to psychotropic drugs. *Dis Nerv Syst* 1961:189–192, 1961.

DERMATOLOGICAL EFFECTS

Photosensitivity

Presentation

There is a sunburnlike erythematous eruption, with or without edema, papules, macules, vesicles, or bullae. The sunburn reaction is usually intense and can be accompanied by blistering, occurring within a few hours of exposure. Lesions are usually confined to exposed areas and subside quickly after withdrawal of the drug or protection from UV (ultraviolet) sources. (Photosensitivity is particularly a consideration for fair-skinned patients.)

Incidence

The incidence is approximately 3%, with chlorpromazine most often implicated.

Mechanism

The reaction is thought to be a phototoxic one caused by the drug itself with free radical formation, or it may be a photoallergic reaction (immunological) resulting from long-wave UV light (320–400 nm). Fluorescent lights are also a source of UV.

Clinical Significance

Many commonly used agents are also photosensitizing agents (thiazides; hypoglycemic agents; antibiotics: tetracycline, sulfonamide; antihistamines: diphenhydramine, promethazine; benzodiazepines: chlordiazepoxide, dibucaine, nalidixic acid; fungicidal creams, medicated soaps; oral contraceptives—estrogen component; cosmetics; and industrial chemicals). Differential diagnosis should also include pellagra, and barbiturate-induced porphyria.

Recommendations

1. Prevent the reaction by educating the patient—advise the patient to wear protective clothing.
2. Instruct the patient to use a sunscreen lotion that contains benzophenone, which protects against the offending UV waves. p-Aminobenzoic acid protects only against middle UV. UVAL® protects against short, middle, and long UV light (260/350 nm); it contains oxybenzone 6%. The lotion must be reapplied during the day, especially between 10:00 A.M. and 4:00 P.M.
3. Rule out other photosensitizers:
   a. A laboratory work-up for porphyrin metabolites in blood, urine, and stool would be helpful.
4. Rule out dermatological conditions exacerbated by anxiety, allergic rashes, and other rare skin reactions (such as angioneurotic edema, exfoliative dermatitis, and Stevens–Johnson syndrome).
5. If the patient is receiving a phenothiazine (particularly chlorpromazine), you may want to recommend changing to another neuroleptic if the photosensitivity reaction is a continuous problem.
6. The addition of diphenhydramine has been claimed to alleviate the burning and itching, as well as the rash.

Pigmentation

Presentation

This reaction usually involves sun-exposed areas. The coloration of the skin has been variously described as a slate gray, bluish-brownish, metallic purple color occurring after years of treatment with phenothiazines. As a comparison, antimalarial agents have been noted to produce a patchy black pigmentation.

Incidence

The incidence was reported as 1% in the 1960s, but pigmentation is rarely found today, which may be related either to the use of drug holidays and current trends to minimize exposure to large doses or to less impurities in the drug formulation. All phenothiazines have been implicated, but chlorpromazine in particular.

Mechanism

Postulated mechanisms include increased melanin formation and blockade of melanocyte-stimulating hormone. The melanosis is considered a phototoxic reaction caused by chlorpromazine or its metabolites.

Clinical Significance

If pigmentation is present, it is also possible that corneal lens opacities exist. The pigmentation is cumulative and may fade during the winter months. The discoloration does not appear to be reversible, even when the drug is discontinued. In one report, 85% of the cases were associated with persons having light brown or brown-gray (salt and pepper) hair color. High doses, long-term therapy, and females appear to be the risk factors for susceptibility to skin pigmentation.

Recommendations

1. Limit the dose and duration of therapy.
2. Switch to another type of neuroleptic (nonphenothiazine).

Suggested Readings

Appleton W. *et al.:* Dermatological effects, in Shader R., DiMascio A. (eds): *Psychotropic Drug Side Effects.* Baltimore, Williams & Wilkins, 1970.

Korwenyi C.: The effects of benzophenone sunscreen lotion on chlor-promazine treated patients. *Am J Psychiatry* 125:143–146, 1969.

Pathak M., Fitzpatrick T.: Photosensitivity caused by drugs. *Rational Drug Ther* 6(6):June 1972.

Rothschild C. T.: Diphenhydramine for phenothiazine-induced photosensitivity. *Can Med Assoc J* 125:1086, 1981.

Satanova A.: Pigmentation due to phenothiazines in high and prolonged dosage. *J Am Med Assoc* 191:87–92, 1965.

Zelickson A.: Skin changes and chlorpromazine—Some hazards of long-term treatment. *J Am Med Assoc* 198:341–344, 1966.

Skin Rashes

Presentation

The rash usually occurs at least 1 week after treatment is initiated. The typical distribution is on the face, trunk, and extremities. It may manifest in various forms—maculopapular rash, urticarial rash, and erythema multiforme.

Incidence

The reaction is probably associated with all neuroleptics, although it is most commonly seen with chlorpromazine. The reported incidence of allergic reaction is 10% of patients on chlorpromazine.

Clinical Significance

The most common type of rash seen is the maculopapular rash, which is benign in nature. Rarely, the patient may develop angioneurotic edema or exfoliative dermatitis, which can be potentially fatal. There is no correlation between the appearance of a rash and the dose of the neuroleptic ingested. The appearance of a rash does *not* mean that the patient will develop an anaphylactic reaction. One must also consider other causes of rash, e.g., food, cosmetics, soap. There may be some cross-sensitivity with other structurally related agents.

Recommendations

1. Discontinuation of treatment is usually unnecessary.
2. If the drug is discontinued, you may restart therapy with the same drug once the rash has subsided without recurrence of the rash, but it might be more prudent to use a structurally unrelated antipsychotic agent.
3. Provide symptomatic relief—antihistamines and topical preparations to alleviate discomfort.

Suggested Readings

Appleton W. S.: The false drug side effect—Which patients complain? *Br J Psychiatry* 114:197–201, 1967.
Baer R. L., Harris H.: Types of cutaneous reactions to drugs. *J Am Med Assoc* 202:710–713, 1967.
Davies D. M.: *Textbook of Adverse Drug Reactions.* New York, Oxford University Press, 1976.
Prien R. F., Cole J. O.: High dose chlorpromazine therapy in chronic schizophrenia. *Arch Gen Psychiatry* 18:482–495, 1968.
Shader R. I., DiMascio A.: *Psychotropic Drug Side Effects.* Baltimore, Williams & Wilkins, 1970.

HEMATOLOGICAL EFFECTS

Agranulocytosis

Presentation

1. Usual onset is within the first 3 months of therapy. Of the cases reported, 90% occur within the first 8 weeks of therapy.
2. Dose and duration of chlorpromazine are important factors.
3. Individual susceptibility is also a factor:
   a. Age—one study reports that 70% of cases of agranulocytosis occur in the age range 40–70 years.
   b. Patients who have impaired marrow function in the absence of the drug are at greater risk.
   c. Females are more frequently involved.

Incidence

Phenothiazine-induced agranulocytosis is a significant blood dyscrasia (alteration in blood cells). Studies with chlorpromazine report a very low incidence of 1 : 250,000 to 1 : 3000–4000 people developing agranulocytosis. The incidence of agranulocytosis is considerably higher with clozapine, from 1 : 10,000 to 2 : 1000. However, clozapine is not used as frequently as other neuroleptics, and the precise incidence is still unknown.

Mechanism

Chlorpromazine-induced agranulocytosis is thought to be caused by a toxic (metabolic)-type reaction or an allergic reaction. The toxic (metabolic) type appears to be dose- and duration-related. The allergic type is believed to occur when the medication combines with the leukocytes, forming an antigenic substance (a substance the body rejects).

Clinical Significance

Frequent blood monitoring is not helpful. If the patient complains of sore throat, malaise, or flu-like symptoms, these may be symptoms of an allergic type of agranulocytosis.

Recommendations

1. Discontinue the drug if leukocytes are less than 3500 mm^3 and neutrophils are less than 30% of total differential.
2. Observe daily if leukocytes are 3500–4000 mm^3 and neutrophils are 30–50% of total differential.
3. Weekly CBC is not reliable in prevention because the onset is sudden.
4. Watch for warning signs (e.g., sore throat, fever).
5. Agranulocytosis may remit if the offending drug is discontinued. Recovery can be seen in 2 weeks and is facilitated if preventive measures against infection (e.g., isolation, antibiotic therapy) are taken. Existing infections should be treated aggressively.
6. Allowing 2 weeks for remission to be complete, it is recommended to change therapy to a different class of neuroleptic drug to prevent the recurrence of agranulocytosis—another phenothiazine (piperazine) or another class of neuroleptic (butyrophenone or thioxanthine).
7. One study suggests calculating the cumulative dosage in susceptible patients. Chlorpromazine-induced agranulocytosis was observed to occur within 20–40

days with a cumulative dose of 10–20 g (500 mg/day).

Suggested Readings

Ananth J. V., Beszterczey A.: Treatment of psychosis subsequent to phenothiazine-induced agranulocytosis. *Comp Psychiatry* 14(4):319–323, 1973.

Ananth J. V., Valles J. V., Whitelaw J. P.: Usual and unusual agranulocytosis during neuroleptic therapy. *Am J Psychiatry* 130(1):100–102, 1973.

Blackburn *et al:* The effects of some drugs which cause agranulocytosis on protein synthesis in human agranulocytes. *Biochem Pharmacol* 24:829–834, 1975.

Litrak R., Kaelblung R.: Agranulocytosis, leukopenia and psychotropic drugs. *Arch Gen Psychiatry* 24:265, 1971.

Marcus J., Mulvilhill F.: Agranulocytosis and chlorpromazine. *J Clin Psychiatry* 39:784–786, 1978.

Pisciotta V.: Drug-induced agranulocytosis. *Drugs* 15:132–143, 1978.

Other Blood Dyscrasias

Presentation

Various hematological abnormalities have been reported, including hemolytic anemia, leukopenia, leukocytosis, neutropenia, and thrombocytopenic purpura (see the preceding section for agranulocytosis).

Incidence

Thrombocytopenia is very rare, but may be more common with phenothiazine antipsychotics.

Mechanism

Although not well understood, these dyscrasias are thought to be a type of allergic or hypersensitivity reaction. In most cases, they are not dose-related, although there is a report of neutropenia following accidental ingestion of 1.5–3 g chlorpromazine by a 5-year-old girl, which implicates a direct toxic effect on bone marrow.

Clinical Significance

Development of any hematological abnormalities requires careful and prompt medical attention. Routine frequent monitoring of blood counts may not always be helpful in identifying problems, since some of these abnormalities develop rapidly over a few days. Transient leukopenia has been more commonly reported, and the situation can be monitored once it develops.

Recommendations

Immediate discontinuation of the suspected offending agent is usually indicated, with close monitoring. Additional medical supervision may be required to provide supportive therapy (e.g., immunosuppressants, prophylactic antibiotics). Should reinstitution of an antipsychotic be necessary after resolution of the hematological abnormality, a chemically unrelated neuroleptic may avoid a recurrence of the problem, although cross-sensitivity has been reported.

Suggested Readings

Burckart G. J. et al: Neutropenia following acute chlorpromazine ingestion. Clin Toxicol 18:797–801, 1981.

Cutler N. R., Heiser J. F.: Leukopenia following treatment with thiothixene and haloperidol. J Am Med Assoc 242:2872–2873, 1979.

Holt R. J.: Neuroleptic drug-induced changes in platelet levels. J Clin Psychopharmacol 4:130–132, 1984.

HEPATIC EFFECTS: JAUNDICE

Presentation

The clinical picture is similar to that of obstructive cholestatic jaundice. Onset is within the first month of treatment; it is usually insidious, but may have a prodrome. The prodromal period (5–7 days) is usually abrupt in onset and may consist of fever, chills, nausea, epigastric or right quandrant abdominal pains, malaise, and rash. The clinical picture does vary; the patient may have mild jaundice with minimal symptoms (fever, abdominal pain, and no jaundice) or abnormal liver function tests and no symptoms.

Laboratory changes are like those in other types of obstructive jaundice: increases in alkaline phosphatase, conjugated bilirubin, BSP retention, SGOT, and eosinophils. Caution should be used not to rely on one single lab test to reach the conclusion of hepatic disease. Abnormalities in liver function tests are seen more frequently than actual clinical jaundice.

With prompt detection, the normal course is usually short and self-limiting. After the drug is discontinued, the condition clears without residual effect in 2–8 weeks.

Incidence

Chlorpromazine is most often implicated. Cross-sensitivity to other phenothiazines is rare. An incidence of 0.5–1% is reported (decreasing in recent years), however, it is as high as 40% on reexposure to a previously offending agent. There is no relationship to age, sex, or dose. Preexisting hepatic disease does not increase susceptibility, but caution should be observed in a patient with severe liver disease.

Case reports have appeared for other phenothiazines (retrospective reports in which the phenothiazine was thought to be the etiology of hepatitis). Large population studies early on with haloperidol revealed a very low incidence, and it was felt that this low incidence is difficult to distinguish from viral hepatitis. Nevertheless, more recently, there have been rare reports of cholestatic liver disease with haloperidol. Other nonphenothiazines implicated are thiothixene, loxapine, and molindone.

Mechanism

The reaction is believed to be a hypersensitivity type of reaction.

Recommendations

1. Discontinue the suspected medication and continue to monitor clinical symptoms and lab data.
2. A chlorpromazine-sensitive patient who is started on another phenothiazine should be carefully monitored, and liver function tests should be performed for 1 month or longer.
3. In patients who are susceptible, the use of haloperidol is recommended.

Suggested Readings

Bassuk E. L.: *The Practitioner's Guide to Psychoactive Drugs*. New York, Plenum Press, 1978, p 99.

Dincsoy H. P., Saelinger D. A.: Haloperidol-induced chronic cholestatic liver disease. *Gastroenterology* 83:694–700, 1982.

Hollister L. E., Hall R. A.: Phenothiazine derivatives and morphologic changes in the liver. *Am J Psychiatry* 123:211–212, 1966.

Ishak K. G., Irey N. S.: Hepatic injury associated with the phenothiazines: Clinicopathologic and followup study of 36 patients. *Arch Pathol* 93:283–304, 1972.

Ponte C. D., Decker E. L.: Leukopenia and hepatotoxicity. *Drug Intell Clin Pharm* 10:562–565, 1976.

Shader R. I.: Hepatic effects, in *Psychotropic Drug Side Effects*. Baltimore, Williams and Wilkins, 1970, pp 175–186.

METABOLIC AND ENDOCRINE EFFECTS

Amenorrhea and Galactorrhea

Presentation

Both amenorrhea and galactorrhea are associated with excessive prolactin secretion. Amenorrhea is defined as an absence of menstruation. Primary amenorrhea is defined as amenorrhea in a patient who has never menstruated; secondary amenorrhea, in a patient who had previously menstruated but has stopped for more than 3 months. The amenorrhea is categorized as psychogenic when there is no identifiable abnormality, often a feature in psychiatric conditions. Galactorrhea is the secretion of milk from the breast at a non-postpartum time. It is frequently, but not always, accompanied by amenorrhea. Any disturbance in the hypothalamic–pituitary axis may result in this syndrome.

All neuroleptics (primarily phenothiazines have been studied) cause endocrine effects based on their mechanism of action. The increase in prolactin helps explain the occurrence of these side effects, but there is no simple relationship between the magnitude of serum prolactin increases and side effects. One report postulated that the variation in prolactin levels may reflect the variation in serum levels of neuroleptics. Tolerance to the increase in prolactin does not develop with long-term administration of the drug. Duration of treatment may not be an important factor, and there may exist a maximal dosage at which the prolactin response maximizes. One must rule out pregnancy, psychogenic causes, organic causes, and the reliability of the patient to report any menstrual disturbance.

Incidence

The reported incidence of galactorrhea is variable (0–80%). Variability may be due to patients not recognizing the galactorrhea and to the different methods used in the studies to ascertain the diagnosis. The general incidence of amenorrhea has been reported to be 3–4%, but in one report, the incidence was noted to be 70%.

Mechanism

Dopamine is believed to be the prolactin-inhibitory factor that is released from the tuberoinfundibular dopamine neurons of the hypothalamus. Dopamine acts on receptors at the pituitary by an unknown mechanism, resulting in decreased prolactin secretion. Interference with dopamine at these receptors will result in increased prolactin secretion.

Recommendations

1. Obtain information from the admission physical examination:
   a. Complete history of menstruation (if at all possible).
   b. Complete drug history including specific medication, dosage, and duration taken prior to admission.
2. One can reduce the dosage or discontinue medication. Individual studies show decreased prolactin levels after withdrawal of medication, although no correlation has been established between the decreased levels and a change in side effects.
3. Serum prolactin levels are easily determined, but since a definite correlation between serum elevations and side effects has not been established, prolactin serum levels are not useful at this time.
4. Use of a dopamine agonist (e.g., bromocriptine) for drug-induced syndromes has not proven useful, and may exacerbate the psychosis.

Suggested Readings

Beumont P., Bruwer J., Pimstone B., *et al:* Bromergocriptine in the treatment of phenothiazine-induced galactorrhoea. *Br J Psychiatry* 126:285–288, 1975.

Frye P. E., Pariser S. F., Kim M. H., *et al:* Bromocriptine associated with symptoms exacerbation during neuroleptic treatment of schizoaffective schizophrenia. *J Clin Psychiatry* 43:252–253, 1982.

Gruen P. H., Sachar E. J., Langer G., *et al:* Prolactin responses to neuroleptics in normal and schizophrenic subjects. *Arch Gen Psychiatry* 35:108–116, 1978.

Kirby R. W., Rotchen T. A., Rees E. D.: Hyperprolactinemia—A review of recent advances. *Arch Intern Med* 139-1415–1419, 1979.

Meltzer H. Y.: Effect of psychotropic drugs on neuroendocrine function. *Psychiatr Clin North Am* 3(2):277–298, 1980.

Meltzer H. Y., Fang V. S.: The effect of neuroleptics on serum prolactin in schizophrenic patients. *Arch Gen Psychiatry* 33:279–286, 1976.

Simpson G. M., Pi E. H., Sramek J. J.: Adverse effects of antipsychotic agents. *Drugs* 21:138–151, 1981.

Appearance of Medication in Breast Milk

Presentation

Neuroleptics that have been reported to be excreted into breast milk include chlorpromazine, trifluoperazine, thioridazine, mesoridazine, haloperidol, piperacetazine, prochlorperazine, and "possibly all phenothiazines." Correlation of dose ingestion with excretion does not yet exist.

Mechanism

Proposed mechanisms include simple diffusion and active transport. Simple diffusion is influenced by the plasma–milk concentration gradient, lipid solubility, and degree of ionization. Other influencing factors include protein-binding characteristics and acid–base characteristics (milk, with a pH of 6.8, tends to collect drugs that are weak bases). Amounts found in breast milk are low (5 mg/ml in breast milk after an average dose of 30 mg of haloperidol).

Clinical Significance

No significant neonatal side effects have been reported. However, it is advisable to avoid breast feeding completely if the patient is taking neuroleptics.

Suggested Readings

Anath B.: Side effects in the neonate from psychotropic agents excreted through breast feeding. *Am J Psychiatry* 135(7):801–805, 1978.

Howard F. M., Hill J. M.: Drugs in pregnancy. *Obstet Gynecol Surv* 34(9):643–653, 1979.

O'Brien T. E.: Excretion of drugs in human milk. *Am J Hosp Pharm* 31(9):844–854, 1974.

Stewart R. B., Karas B., Springer P.: Haloperidol excretion in human milk. *Am J Psychiatry* 137(7)849–850, 1980.

Gynecomastia

Presentation

The patient may complain of breast tenderness and swelling.

Incidence

Occurrence is uncommon; therefore, the clinician must rule out other causes for the gynecomastia. No information is available to determine which neuroleptic is more prone to cause gynecomastia.

Mechanism

Gynecomastia may occur from an increased secretion of luteotropic hormone affecting the mammary tissue or from effects of increased gonadotropic hormone on the production of estrogen by the testes.

Recommendations

If the neuroleptic is the suspected agent, discontinue use or lower the dosage.

Suggested Readings

Beumong P. J., Gelder M. G., Friesen H. G., *et al:* The effects of phenothiazines on endocrine function. *Br J Psychiatry* 124:413, 1974.
Margolis I. B., Gross C. G.: Gynecomastia during phenothiazine therapy. *J Am Med Assoc* 41:942–944, 1967.

Hyperglycemia

Presentation

Chlorpromazine causes a slight but statistically significant increase in blood glucose levels. The mild transient increase usually remits when the drug is withdrawn.

Mechanism

The mechanism is not known, but hyperglycemia is believed to be due to increased release of catecholamines from the adrenals.

Recommendations

Psychotropic agents are not contraindicated in patients who have diabetes mellitus, but one needs to be aware of the potential of altered glucose handling. Monitor serum glucose levels when using neuroleptic medication, especially in diabetics.

Suggested Reading

Earle G., Bass M.: Effect of chlorpromazine on blood glucose and plasma insulin in man. *Eur J Clin Psychopharmacol* 11:15–18, 1977.

Placental Transfer

Mechanism

Proposed mechanisms include simple diffusion, active transport, pinocytosis, leakage, placental metabolism of drug, and modification of the permeability of the placental barrier (due to an interaction of the drug molecule with cell membrane structures). The major mechanism is simple diffusion.

The most significant factors that influence diffusion include lipid solubility (greater transfer with increased lipid solubility) and molecular size (greater transfer with smaller molecular size). A molecular weight of greater than 1000 is relatively impermeable; a weight of less than 600 is readily permeable. Other factors include pH, pKa, area of maternal–fetal exchange, thickness of the membranes drugs must pass, rate of maternal–placental blood flow, and free drug concentration. Detectable concentrations of all psychotropics have been reported in fetal circulation.

There are case reports of parent drug and metabolites found in fetal/neonate plasma, urine, and/or amniotic fluid. Newborns may experience side effects, since neuroleptics have been reported to pass into the fetal circulation. There have been reports of extrapyramidal effects caused by phenothiazines. These symptoms are invariably transient and respond to diphendyramine (5 mg/kg per day). Neonatal jaundice and hyperbilirubinemia have been reported in newborns of phenothiazine-treated mothers. Many cases were reported in premature infants (low birth weight). Melanin deposits have also been reported. The majority of cases claim negative effects, and no correlation between neuroleptic use and jaundice has been established.

Suggested Readings

Hammond J. E., and Toseland P. A.: Placental transfer of chlorpromazine. *Arch Dis Child* 45:139–140, 1970.

Fedelina O'Donoghue S. E.: Distribution of pethidine and chlorpromazine in maternal, fetal and neonatal biological fluids. *Nature (London)* 229:124–125, 1971.

Sexual Dysfunction

Presentation

Psychiatric disorders are frequently associated with alteration in sexual behavior and function, including decreased libido, inability to reach orgasm, difficulty in maintaining an erection, decreased vaginal lubrication, and retrograde ejaculation.

Incidence

The incidence of sexual dysfunction appears to be higher with thioridazine and with medications with similar side effects, such as mesoridazine and chlorpromazine. In addition, all neuroleptics cause sedation and may contribute to increasing the incidence of sexual dysfunction.

Mechanism

This group of medications affects sexual function by altering the activity of the autonomic nervous and tuboinfundibular systems of the CNS. Specifically, the parasympathetic is responsible for erection and may cause or contribute to inhibited sexual excitement. The sympathetic nervous system is responsible for ejaculation and may cause or exacerbate premature orgasm or inhibited male orgasm. These effects on the CNS by neuroleptics may contribute to alteration in the desire phase of sexual function for both males and females.

Recommendations

1. Define the nature of the sexual dysfunction.
2. Rule out functional vs. organic causes.
3. Change to another class of neuroleptic, with low anticholinergic properties, if the problem persists.
4. Reassure the patient that these effects are not harmful and are reversible.

Suggested Readings

Buffum J.: Pharmacosexology: The effects of drugs on sexual function—A review. *J Psychoactive Drugs* 14:1–2, 1982.

Federman D.: Impotence: Etiology and management. *Hosp Pract,* March 1982.

Horowitz J. *et al:* Drugs and impaired male sexual function. *Drugs* 18, 1979.

Munjack D. J., Oziel J. L.: *Sexual Medicine and Counseling in Office Practice.* Boston, Little, Brown, 1980.

Shen V.: Thioridazine-induced inhibition of female orgasm. *Psychiatr J Univ Ottawa* 7(4), 1982.

Weight Gain

Incidence

The incidence of weight gain is not precisely known and may be more common with low-potency neuroleptics (e.g., chlorpromazine) than with high-potency neuroleptics (e.g., haloperidol). All neuroleptics have been implicated in causing weight gain with the possible exception of molindone (Moban®). However, a recent study has not found this to be the case.

Mechanism

The mechanism is not known precisely. The following mechanisms have been suggested:
1. Increased fluid intake and retention:
   a. Rapid weight gain early in therapy.
   b. Increased intake of fluids, which may be due to dry mouth.
   c. Increase in ACTH and antidiuretic hormone (ADH).
   d. Increased intake of high-calory drinks, e.g., soft drinks.
2. Increased appetite and carbohydrate craving:
   a. Increased availability of food (often high in carbo-hydrates) during hospitalization.
   b. Patients report a "carbohydrate craving."
   c. Resolution of psychosis—appetite returns to normal.
3. Anticholinergic potency:
   a. Noted weight gain associated with thioridazine and chlorpromazine.
   b. Side effect of "dry mouth" may lead to increased fluid intake.
4. Altered glucose monitoring activity of hypothalamus and glucose tolerance.
5. Decreased motor activity:
   a. Restricted ward environment.
   b. Sedative action of the extrapyramidal symptoms due to neuroleptics.
   c. Fat deposition or redistribution.

Clinical Significance

1. Factors other than medication may be involved (individual tendency to gain weight must be considered).
2. Weight gain may interfere with compliance. Some

40–50% of outpatients discontinue medications, a common reason being weight gain.

3. Molindone and loxapine are possibly associated with no weight change, but one recent study reported weight gain with molindone.
4. Weight gain is usually reversible and most often occurs with long-term therapy.
5. Further investigation is definitely needed.

Recommendations

1. Educate the patient concerning the role of diet and exercise in weight gain.
2. Increase physical activity.
3. Decrease caloric intake.
4. Clinical evidence exists that switching from one phenothiazine to another will sometimes reduce the weight-gaining tendency without interfering with the antipsychotic activity.

Suggested Readings

Branchey M., Simpson G.: High and low-potency neuroleptics in elderly psychotic patients. *J Am Med Assoc* 239:1860–1862, 1978.

Earle G., Bass M.: Effect of chlorpromazine on blood glucose and plasma insulin in man. *Eur J Clin Pharmacol* 11:15–18, 1977.

Parent M. M., Roy S., Sramek J., *et al:* Effect of molindone on weight change in hospitalized schizophrenic patients. *Drug Intell Clin Pharm* 20:873–875, 1986.

Breast Cancer

Presentation

There has been concern that neuroleptic use may increase the possibility of developing breast cancer in females.

Incidence

Studies have failed to demonstrate an association between neuroleptics and an increased likelihood of breast cancer.

Mechanism

Breast cancer is postulated to result from increased prolactin levels caused by neuroleptics. There has also been postulation that long-term neuroleptic treatment may cause pituitary tumors, but this has not been substantiated by investigation.

Clinical Significance

Since an association among neuroleptics, prolactin, and breast cancer has not been shown, most experts believe there is no reason for concern. However, it would be best to avoid neuroleptics in a high-risk female with a known prolactin-dependent tumor. The future availability of neuroleptic drugs that do not elevate prolactin (e.g., clozapine) will obviate any such concerns.

Suggested Readings

Lilford V. A. *et al:* Long-term phenothiazine treatment does not cause
    pituitary tumors. *Br J Psychiatry* 144:421–424, 1984.
Overall J. E.: Breast cancer and treatment with neuroleptics. *Arch Gen
    Psychiatry* 36:604–605, 1979.
Schyue P. M., Smithline F., Meltzer H. Y.: Neuroleptic-induced prolactin
    level elevation and breast cancer. *Arch Gen Psychiatry* 35:1291–1299,
    1978.

NEUROLEPTIC MALIGNANT SYNDROME

Presentation

In full-blown neuroleptic malignant syndrome (NMS), one sees neurological signs (rigidity, akinesia, dyskinesia), high temperature, autonomic dysfunction (increased blood pressure, increased heart rate, sweating); the mental status can range from obtundation to coma. The NMS is usually seen within 2 weeks of initiating antipsychotic treatment, but there have been cases of late onset reported (up to years later). NMS evolves over the course of 1–3 days and lasts from 5 to 10 days except in the event that long-acting depot neuroleptics are involved. In such cases, the course of NMS may last 2–3 times longer. Laboratory results are helpful in NMS, but not always specific; these include leukocytosis (with left shift), increased creatine phosphokinase (CPK) of muscle origin, also sometimes increased liver enzymes, and slowing in the electroencephalogram (EEG).

Incidence

Once thought to be very rare (around 0.5%), NMS may be of higher incidence today because of better recognition and awareness of the syndrome. Younger males are most often affected, and high-potency neuroleptics such as haloperidol and fluphenazine have been most often implicated. Patients with affective disorders may be more predisposed to development of NMS.

Mechanism

NMS is thought to result from the central blockade of dopamine receptors in the hypothalamus and possibly the nigrostriatum, but this does not appear to be a full explanation of NMS, and a molecular mechanism involving intracellular calcium may underlie or modulate the effects on the dopamine system that trigger NMS.

Clinical Significance

There is a high reported incidence of mortality in NMS (approximately 20%); therefore, prevention of NMS assumes real importance. If NMS is suspected, prompt treatment measures should be instituted. Treatment should be especially geared to vigilance in preventing any medical complications such as pneumonia, cardiovascular collapse, or pulmonary embolus. Some of these complications may arise from the ridigity and immobilization brought about by neuroleptics in susceptible patients and would thus represent untreated or unrecognized consequences of severe neurological reactions of the extrapyramidal type.

Recommendations

When one suspects NMS, the condition should be differentiated from other conditions such as catatonia, akinetic mutism, hyperthermia (drug-induced, malignant hyperthermia), or other neurotoxic reactions involving therapeutic drugs or drugs of abuse. Promptly discontinue neuroleptics and institute supportive treatment, including (when needed) cooling, increasing fluids, electrolytes, and preventive measures against infections. A thorough medical work-up should be done to rule out other conditions. If symptoms are mild and involve primarily severe forms of extrapyramidal reactions, these should be treated with antiparkinson agents, but care should be taken because these drugs also interfere with temperature regulation and can add to the increased temperature. Other agents that have been claimed to be helpful include benzodiazepines, amantadine, bromocriptine, L-dopa, dantrolene, calcium-channel blockers, and β-blockers; the success of these treatments is, however, only empirical.

Suggested Readings

Abbott R. J., Loizou L. A.: Neuroleptic malignant syndrome. *Br J Psychiatry* 148:47–51, 1986.

Berkimer L. J., DeVane C. L.: The neuroleptic malignant syndrome: Presentation and treatment. *Drug Intell Clin Pharm* 18:462–465, 1984.

Caroff S. N.: The neuroleptic malignant syndrome. *J Clin Psychiatry* 41:79–83, 1980.

Hashimoto F. *et al:* Neuroleptic malignant syndrome and dopaminergic blockade. *Arch Intern Med* 144:629–630, 1984.

Levinson D. F., Simpson G. M.: Neuroleptic-induced extrapyramidal symptoms with fever. *Arch Gen Psychiatry* 43:839–848, 1986.

Mueller P. S., Vester J. W., Fermaglich J.: Neuroleptic malignant
    syndrome. *J Am Med Assoc* 249(3):386–388, 1983.

NEUROLOGICAL EFFECTS

Anticholinergic Psychosis

Presentation

The time of onset varies; it may be several hours or
much later into the treatment. A variety of symptoms have
been reported:

Central effects: disorientation, confusion, hallucinations
(usually visual, but can be auditory, tactile, or all three),
delusions, memory loss, agitation, dysarthria, incoherent or
pressured speech, ataxia, fluctuating mental status, coma.
Severe impairment of recent memory is a prominent feature
of intoxication.

Peripheral effects: widely dilated and poorly reactive
pupils, blurred vision, warm dry skin, flushed face, decreased secretions of the mouth, pharynx, nose, and bronchi,
foul breath, fever, tachycardia, elevated blood pressure, decreased bowel activity, hyperreflexia, urinary retention, and
increased respiratory rate. The most consistent physiological
signs are those of peripheral muscarinic blockade, particularly
dilated and poorly reactive pupils.

Incidence

Anticholinergic psychosis has been reported in patients
on neuroleptics, antiparkinson agents, and tricyclic antidepressants, either alone or in combination. Confusional
states are often produced in elderly patients, who are particularly sensitive to the central anticholinergic effects of drugs.

Mechanism

The syndrome arises from the competitive inhibition of
acetylcholine by atropinelike substances at central and pe-

ripheral cholinergic muscarinic sites. When neuroleptics, anticholinergics, and antidepressants are used in combination, the
anticholinergic effects are believed to be additive or
potentiated.

Clinical Significance

The diagnosis may be difficult to differentiate from a
worsening of the patient's primary psychotic state; however,
the combination of both central and peripheral symptoms
gives a relatively specific picture for anticholinergic psychosis. One must always rule out other drug intoxications
(hallucinogens, cannabis, PCP, alcohol, narcotics), which
may exhibit a similar or different clinical picture depending
on the drug ingested. Death due to anticholinergic intoxication is rare. A fatality may occur indirectly when the
delirious patient is uncontrollable and may harm himself.

Recommendations

1. Discontinue the offending agent.
2. Conduct a careful physical examination, ECG, lab
   work-up, and mental status evaluation to determine
   definite diagnosis.
3. Patients should be hospitalized to:
   a. Prevent accidental injury to themselves or others.
   b. Control hyperthermia.
   c. Minimize fluctuations in vital signs.
   d. Institute cardiac monitoring.
4. In many cases of anticholinergic psychosis, observa-
   tion and reassurance are all that is needed.
5. To control agitation, diazepam can be given, 5–12.5
   mg either orally or parenterally (IV), if a quicker
   onset is desired. Phenothiazines, especially thioridazine and chlorpromazine, should not be used to
   treat agitation, since they can exacerbate the intoxication due to their anticholinergic activity.
6. Physostigmine is used if the patient is exhibiting
   classic symptoms (increased temperature, delirium,

agitation, or coma). A cholinesterase inhibitor is useful for supraventricular tachyarrhythmias, then administer antiarrhythmics such as lidocaine, phenytoin, or propanolol, if indicated.

Suggested Readings

Bluhm R. E., Koller W. C.: Anticholinergic abuse—when to suspect it, what to do about it. *Drug Ther* 1981:150–155, 1981.

Heiser M., Gilli J. C.: The reversal of anticholinergic drug induced delirium and coma with physostigmine. *Am J Psychiatry* 127:1050–1054, 1971.

Johnson A. L., Hollister L. E., Berger P. A.: The anticholinergic intoxication syndrome: Diagnosis and treatment. *Am J Psychiatry* 42(8):313–317, 1981.

Lang A. W., Moore R. A.: Acute toxic psychosis concurrent with phenothiazine therapy. *Am J Psychiatry* 128:95–99, 1971.

Snyder D. L., Greenberg D., Yamamura H. I.: Antischizophrenic drugs and brain cholinergic receptors. *Arch Gen Psychiatry* 31:58–61, 1974.

Extrapyramidal Symptoms

Mechanism

Dopamine blocking of neuroleptics in the nigrostriatal tract is felt to be the etiology of the extrapyramidal symptoms (EPS). The result is a relative cholinergic predominance with the emergence of EPS.

Presentation, Incidence, and Clinical Significance

The appearance of EPS is most commonly seen with the high-potency neuroleptics, such as haloperidol and fluphenazine.

Dystonic reaction: bizarre, involuntary contractions of muscles, primarily in the neck and head (mouth, tongue), but also in the back, arms, and legs. The onset is usually at the initiation of therapy, within 24–48 hr. It is thought to be more prevalent in young males. The types of dystonia seen include the following: head—oculogyric crisis (eyes are turned in an upward gaze), facial grimacing, spasm of the tongue and mouth, possibly some difficulty in speaking, drooling; neck musculature—torticollis (head and neck twisted to one side); back—opisthotonus (arched back); extremities—arm and leg stiffness, arms may appear slightly flexed and rigid, leg stiffness may produce bizarre gaits, some difficulty with motor dexterity. There are also rare reports of persistent dystonia (tardive dystonia), which is very difficult to treat.

Akathisia: subjective feeling of inner restlessness, muscle discomfort, a need or desire to be in constant motion. The onset is usually within the first few weeks of therapy. Many patients may have difficulties describing their feelings of restlessness and may associate these feelings with fright, anxiety, or irritability. Akathisia can present as pacing, having difficulty falling asleep, or not being able to sit still. It is necessary to differentiate akathisia from the psychotic state (although the differentiation is difficult to make) to avoid increasing the neuroleptic dose, which may further exacerbate the condition.

Pseudoparkinsonism: The onset is usually within several weeks to months after the initiation of therapy. It is stated to be more common in females above 45 years of age. The presentation of symptoms is very similar to that of idiopathic parkinsonism. The masklike face is a loss of facial expression, often with some drooling present. The tremor usually occurs at rest and involves the upper extremities. A general impairment of motor activity occurs as a result of muscle rigidity. This impairment will manifest as the ''Parkinson stance,'' shuffling gait, and akinesia (slowness in initiating movement, and fatigue).

Recommendations

1. Adjust the dose of neuroleptic downward if possible.

2. Switch to an agent with a lower incidence of EPS (e.g., low-potency neuroleptics).
3. Wait for the appearance of EPS before initiating anticholinergic agents.
4. Some clinicians choose to give anticholinergic agents prophylactically to guard against the possibility of developing EPS. There is some evidence proving the efficacy of prophylactic treatment, particularly for the acute dystonias.
5. Treatment with anticholinergic agents should be necessary only for a period of 2–3 months. Of the patients who are treated with an anticholinergic agent for several months, 60% are free of symptoms when the antiparkinson agent is withdrawn. Recommended daily doses for treating extrapyramidal symptoms:

	Adult Dose/Day	Elderly Dose/Day
Benztropine (Cogentin)	1–8 mg PO	1–4 mg PO
	1–8 mg IM/IV*	1–3 mg IM/IV
Trihexyphenidyl (Artane)	2–15 mg PO	2–6 mg PO

Diphenhydramine (Benadryl) has also been used to treat drug-induced EPS. It can be used both orally and parenterally. The dosage range is approximately 25–150 mg/day PO or 25–50 mg IM/IV in divided doses.

6. A few recent reports claim that amantadine and propranolol may be more effective than the aforementioned anticholinergic agents in the treatment of akathisia.

Suggested Readings

Freedman D. X.: American College of Neuropsychopharmacology–Food and Drug Administration task force: Neurological syndromes associated with antipsychotic drug use. *Arch Gen Psychiatry* 28:463–467, 1973.

Goetz C. G., Klawans H. L.: Drug-induced extrapyramidal disorders—A neuropsychiatric interface. *J Clin Psychopharmacol* 1(5):297–303, 1981.

*For acute severe dystonic reactions.

Lipinski J. F. *et al:* Propranolol in the treatment of neuroleptic-induced akathisia. *Am J Psychiatry* 141:412–413, 1984.

Sovner R., DiMascio A.: Extrapyramidal syndromes and other neurological side effects of psychotropic drugs, in Lipton M. A., DiMascio A. (eds): *Psychopharmacology: A Generation of Progress.* New York, Raven Press, 1978, pp 1021–1032.

Sramek J. J., Simpson G. M., Morrison R. L., *et al:* Anticholinergic agents for prophylaxis of neuroleptic-induced dystonic reaction: A perspective study. *J Clin Psychiatry* 47:305–306, 1986.

Psychotic Exacerbation Induced by Neuroleptics

Cases are usually in conjunction with rapid dosage increases, with initiation of new medication after drug holiday, or with higher-dosage regimens. The actual incidence is not known, and the condition is considered a rare phenomenon.

Case reports of psychotic exacerbation indicate that the condition is responsive to discontinuation or decrease in dosage of neuroleptic:

Three cases characterized by repetitive, importunate, infantile, histrionic behavior mixed with a psychotic picture (overactive, excited, assaultive, hallucinations, delusions).

A case described in which haloperidol caused an exacerbation of the psychotic state, the patient becoming more agitated and restless, and an increase in auditory–visual hallucinations and delusions. The symptoms showed marked improvement when the neuroleptic was discontinued. The author felt that the exacerbation was an idiosyncratic response to the neuroleptic and might have been related to an elevated serum level.

Case reports of psychotic exacerbation responsive to parenteral antiparkinson agents:

Description of a general overaroused picture, either inhibited and negativistic or excited and agitated (some situations similar to mute catatonia or catatonic excitement). The use of antiparkinson agents resolved all the aforedescribed behavior.

Other authors have reported similar clinical presentations and have postulated (1) a relationship between a phenothiazine psychosis and an induced sensory deprivation and

(2) a relationship between schizophrenia and EPS (catatonia originating from the nuclei of the extrapyramidal tract). One author described a syndrome with a high-potency neuroleptic marked by features of catatonia that has a gradual onset and responds slowly to withdrawal of the neuroleptic or to addition of an anticholinergic drug and that may be easily confused with worsening of the schizophrenic symptoms.

Recommendations

1. Decrease the neuroleptic dosage.
2. Evaluate for possible akathisia.
3. Discontinue all neuroleptics while the patient is hospitalized and observe for improvement in condition over the next 2–3 days.

Suggested Readings

Ereshefsky L., Davis C. M., Harrington C. A., et al: Haloperidol and reduced haloperidol plasma levels in select schizophrenic patients. *J Clin Psychopharmacol* 4:138–142, 1984.

Magliozzi J. R. et al: Relationship of serum haloperidol levels to clinical response in schizophrenic patients. *Am J Psychiatry* 138(3):365–367, 1981.

Miller D. D., Hersey L. A., Duffy P. J., et al: Serum haloperidol concentration and clinical response in acute psychosis. *J Clin Psychopharmacol* 4:305–310, 1984.

Simpson G. et al.: Psychotic exacerbations produced by neuroleptics. *Dis Nerv Sys* 37(7):367–369, 1976.

Tornatore F., Lee D., Sramek J.: Psychotic exacerbation with haloperidol. *Drug Intell Clin Pharm* 15:209–213, 1981.

Seizure Threshold Alteration

Mechanism

Proposed mechanisms of action—physiological:

1. Suppression of the desynchronization effect of afferent sensory influences on cortical discharges.

2. Decreased amounts of glutamic acid and γ-amino-butyric acid found in brain slices from epileptogenic areas (human and animal) after induced seizure with phenothiazines.
3. Vitamin B_{12} and folate deficiency—it is suggested that anticonvulsant therapy or disturbance in folic acid and vitamin B_{12} may be contributing factors.
4. Imbalance of dopaminergic and cholinergic transmission (based on animal studies and case reports):
    a. Supported by reports of thioridazine and chlorpromazine (high anticholinergic properties) causing seizures in epileptic patients.
    b. Trifluoperazine (weak anticholinergic) does not lower seizure threshold and haloperidol (weaker anticholinergic, potent dopamine blockade) has been reported to have little effect on seizure.

Incidence

Incidence of seizures for chlorpromazine (CPZ) has been reported in dosage groups (no information provided if the population had an existing seizure disorder):

Low Moderate Dose	Incidence
400–800 mg CPZ/day	Less than 0.5%
30–900 mg CPZ/day	0.3 – 5%

High Dose	Incidence
1000–2000 mg CPZ/day	10%
Over 1000 mg CPZ/day	31 – 51%

Presentation

Neuroleptics have been reported to cause diffuse slowing of EEG activity (nonpathological). Drug-induced EEG changes are usually transient, but may persist for weeks after the drug is discontinued.

Clinical Significance

Neuroleptics can induce EEG abnormalities without the occurrence of seizures. Seizures induced by neuroleptics are considered rare and affect fewer than 1% of those taking these drugs.

Aliphatic phenothiazines are considered more epileptogenic compared to other agents. The ability of CPZ to induce seizures is supported by experimental data and is not based purely on the fact that it is more frequently used.

Factors that may contribute to inducing seizures:

1. Large dosages.
2. Sudden dosage changes.
3. Pathology present—Organic Brain Syndrome (OBS), existing seizure disorder.
4. Existing EEG irregularities.
5. Abrupt withdrawal of neuroleptics.
6. Sedating properties of the drug.

Recommendations

1. Avoid sudden dosage changes; an abrupt increase or decrease in dose may precipitate seizures.
2. Avoid combination therapy with more than one neuroleptic drug. This type of therapy may increase seizure susceptibility.
3. Patients with epileptiform manifestations or OBS should be treated more cautiously with psychotropics.
4. Chlorpromazine and thioridazine may not be the drug of choice in seizure-prone patients.
5. Butyrophenone and piperazine phenothiazine are reported to be associated with a decreased incidence of seizures.
6. Be aware of conditions that may further lower the convulsive threshold in a patient on neuroleptics:

hyperglycemia, exhaustion, sudden discontinuance of medication, hyperpyrexia.

7. If the patient is receiving anticonvulsants, psychotic symptoms may be secondary to anticonvulsant toxicity. Verification of toxicity should be made with serum levels; if toxicity is present, treatment involves decreasing or changing the anticonvulsant rather than adding another antipsychotic.

8. If a previously controlled seizure disorder is disturbed in a patient on antipsychotic medication, rather than lower or discontinue the antipsychotic, one may consider increasing the dose of anticonvulsant. In a patient without a history of a seizure disorder who has an isolated seizure (spontaneous), change to another antipsychotic before considering treatment with an anticonvulsant.

9. Competition of metabolic pathways may occur when giving both antipsychotic and anticonvulsant medications. There may be an increase or decrease in the level of either drug; therefore, be aware of possible toxicity, resistance to therapy, or exacerbation of previously controlled seizures.

Suggested Readings

Itil T. M., Sodatos C.: Epileptogenic side effects of psychotropic drugs. *J Am Med Assoc J* 224(13):1460–1463, 1980.

Logothetis J.: Spontaneous epileptic seizures and electroencephalographic changes in the course of phenothiazine therapy. *Neurology* 17:869–877, 1967.

Mendez M. F., Cummings J. L., Benson D. F.: Epilepsy: Psychiatric aspects and use of psychotropics. *Psychosomatics* 25(12):86–93, 1984.

Oliver P. A., Luchins D. J., Wyatt R. J.: Neuroleptic-induced seizures. *Arch Gen Psychiatry* 39:206–209, 1982.

Remick R. A., Fine S. H.: Antipsychotic drugs and seizures. *J Clin Psychiatry* 4:78–80, 1979.

Schlichter W. *et al.:* Seizures occurring during intensive chlorpromazine therapy. *Can Med Assoc* 74:364–392, 1968.

Supersensitivity Psychosis

Presentation

There is a worsening of the psychosis (delusions, hallucinations, suspiciousness) induced by long-term use of neuroleptic drugs. Typically, those who develop supersensitivity psychosis respond well initially to low or moderate doses of antipsychotics, but with time seem to require larger doses after each relapse and ultimately megadoses to control symptoms.

Incidence

Experts debate the existence of supersensitivity psychosis. At present, it is considered uncommon, and there are only a dozen or so cases documented in the literature.

Mechanism

The mechanism is postulated to be receptor supersensitivity to dopamine in the mesolimbic system.

Clinical Significance

If supersensitivity psychosis does exist, then, as with its counterpart, tardive dyskinesia (see the next section), the treatment may be difficult and the syndrome may be irreversible. Supersensitivity psychosis may be difficult to detect because the onset is insidious. If the syndrome is masked by neuroleptic medication, it will appear only on discontinuation of neuroleptic medication or will be manifested by the need for higher doses following a relapse.

Recommendations

Prevention is the best treatment. It is helpful to follow normal dosage guidelines for neuroleptics unless the history or circumstances or both dictate otherwise. The efficacy of high-dose neuroleptic treatment in refractory patients appears less promising than was once thought. If supersensitivity psychosis develops, alternative treatments may be considered, including use of benzodiazepines at higher dosages as well as the use of lithium, which has been shown in animals to assist in the desensitization of receptors.

Suggested Readings

Chouinard G., Jones B. D.: Neuroleptic-induced supersensitivity psychosis: Clinical and pharmacologic characteristics. *Am J Psychiatry* 137:16–21, 1980.

Weinberger D. R. *et al.*: Drug withdrawal in chronic schizophrenic patients: In search of neuroleptic-induced supersensitivity psychosis. *J Clin Psychopharmacol* 1:120–123, 1981.

Tardive Dyskinesia

Presentation

The early description included the classic "BLM" (buccolingual masticatory) triad: involuntary movements of the tongue and lips and chewing movements of the jaw. The current description has expanded to include additional movements: choreoathetoid movements of the fingers, wrist, ankles, and toes; ballistic movements of the upper extremities; axial hyperkinesia; rocking movements; diaphragmatic involvement, grunting; facial grimacing; blinking, tremor of the eyelids, pouting, puckering smack of the lips; and choreoathetoid movements of the tongue. The oral–facial dyskinesias are most common in adults, whereas movements of the extremities are seen more often in children. Usually, the movements increase with stress and disappear during sleep.

Incidence

The reported incidence ranges from 0.5 to 60% in patients treated with prolonged neuroleptic therapy. Studies that do not define the diagnostic criteria used may reflect inaccurate figures; i.e., overinclusive criteria or inclusion of mild dyskinesia will result in higher prevalence, while selection of only severe cases will result in low figures. Most of the current studies find a prevalence rate of 25–30%.

Elderly females have been shown to have a higher incidence of tardive dyskinesia (TD) than males. The total amount of neuroleptic administered over the years appears to have no significant relationship to development of TD, but those who receive higher daily doses over a long period of time may be prone to develop TD. An increased incidence of TD in patients treated with anticholinergic agents and/or in those with a history of neuroleptic-induced EPS has not been firmly established. Senile dyskinesias have been noted in elderly patients who never received neuroleptic, with two studies reporting prevalence rates of 9 and 37%.

Mechanism

The most widely accepted theory about tardive dyskinesia involves the hypothesis of dopamine hypersensitivity. Accordingly, TD results from receptor changes induced by long-term neuroleptic treatment.

Clinical Significance

Differential diagnosis must be considered, including Huntington's chorea, Gilles de la Tourette's syndrome, psychotic mannerism of sterotypic behavior, Wilson's disease, heavy-metal intoxication, systemic metabolic disorders, and many more.

Two subtypes of TD have been described: persistent and withdrawal. Withdrawal TD is the appearance or worsening of symptoms after discontinuance of a neuroleptic (usually high dosages). The condition with either reverse or remission rate improve over time range of 0–90% has been reported after drug withdrawal. In view of this wide range, it is not possible at this time to predict the reversibility of TD.

Drug holidays: Initially, this concept was thought to help prevent development of TD, but it was found that large doses and holidays of 2 months or more were found to contribute to TD. The status of drug holidays is at present controversial.

Recommendations

Various pharmacological measures have been tried without significant results:

1. Dopamine (DA) antagonists: The improvements in symptoms (a masking effect) may be temporary and the condition may worsen (to cause further receptor sensitivity, i.e., to neuroleptics).
2. DA-depleting agents: These agents were thought to deplete DA stores, yet not cause further receptor sensitivity (not yet proven). Some agents were found to produce only temporary improvement, i.e., reserpine and tetrabenazine.
3. Cholinergic agents are thought to have the greatest potential for improving TD. Physostigmine has been reported to lead to improvements, but the parenteral route limits its usefulness. Oral alternatives are available, but the efficacy is questionable, i.e., choline, deanol, lecithin (phosphatidylcholine).
4. γ-Aminobutyric acid agonists are thought to exert an inhibitory effect on the DA system; there are conflicting results in many reports, i.e., benzodiazepines, baclofen, valproic acid, and muscimol.
5. Many miscellaneous agents are used: estrogens, papaverine, propranolol, isocarboxazid, barbiturates, lithium, tryptophan, fusaric acid, and disulfiram.

Prevention

1. Administer a neuroleptic only when clearly indicated.
2. Keep the neuroleptic dosage as low as possible and reevaluate the need for continued neuroleptic therapy (recommended every 3 months).
3. Avoid long-term use of anticholinergics, since their role in TD has not yet been established.
4. Evaluate the patient for signs of TD:
   a. AIMS (Abnormal Involuntary Movement Scores) is an easy-to-use, quick method.
   b. TDRS (Tardive Dyskinesia Rating Scale) or abbreviated version (ADS) by Simpson.

The management of a diagnosed or suspected case of TD

is difficult. The approach to treatment depends on whether a neuroleptic is needed to control the psychiatric symptoms. If the psychiatric condition permits, one may choose to decrease the neuroleptic dose to the lowest effective dose. This is done by gradually withdrawing the neuroleptic, one third of the total dose per month. If the patient is also receiving an antiparkinson agent, this agent too should be withdrawn over a 2- to 3-week period. One must remember that withdrawal dyskinesia from the neuroleptic may appear. For mild dyskinetic symptoms, temporary use of a muscle relaxant or a benzodiazepine (diazepam 20–40 mg) may be helpful. (If the psychotic symptoms are severe, one may need to restart the neuroleptic until the symptoms are controlled.) Haloperidol may be preferred to other neuroleptics (starting at 2 mg/day and increasing approximately every 2 weeks for control of symptoms), because this drug is a purer DA blocker with minimal anticholinergic effects. However, the choice of neuroleptic should be based on past response and compliance.

Suggested Readings

Branchey M., Branchey L.: Patterns of psychotropic drug use and tardive dyskinesia. *J Clin Psychopharmacol* 4:41–45, 1984.

Glazer W., Moore D., Schooler N., et al: Tardive dyskinesia. *Arch Gen Psychiatry* 41:623–627, 1984.

Gualtieri C. T., Barnill J., McGimsey J., et al: Tardive dyskinesia and other movement disorders in children treated with psychotropic drugs. *J Am Acad Child Psychiatry* 19:491–510, 1980.

Jeste D., Wyatt R.: In search of treatment of tardive dyskinesia: Review of the literature. *Schizophr Bull* 5(2):251–293, 1979.

Klawans H., Goetz C., Perlik S.: Tardive dyskinesia: Review and update. *Am J Psychiatry* 137:900–908, 1980.

Simpson G. M., Lee J. H., Zoubok B., Gardos G.: A rating scale for tardive dyskinesia. *Psychopharmacology* 64:171–179, 1979.

Simpson G. M., Pi E. H., Sramek J. J.: Management of tardive dyskinesia: Current update. *Drugs* 23:381–393, 1982.

OCULAR ABNORMALITIES

Corneal Lesions

Presentation

White to yellow-brown granules appear in the cornea. When severe, the lesion may be seen as a slightly brown haze only with the use of a focused light. Deep lesions (endothelium, posterior surface) are usually associated with lens deposits.

Recommendations

Decrease the dose or change to a nonphenothiazine neuroleptic.

Epithelial Keratopathy

This reaction involves the epithelium and the portion of the cornea exposed to light; it is not necessarily associated with lens changes.

Presentation

White, brown, or gray opacities may appear. Linear and curvilinear radiations appear in the lower part of the cornea. The opacities are visible with a slit lamp.

Incidence

The incidence is dose-related (high daily dose, not cumulative dose). Lesions can appear within months of chlopromazine, 2 g/day. Lesions are generally seen with chlorpromazine, and the other phenothiazines are suspected.

Mechanism

The mechanism is unknown, but the position of the lesion suggests a dermatological-related form of photosensitivity.

Clinical Significance

The lesion does not significantly impair visual acuity. It is partially reversible on discontinuation of the neuroleptic.

Recommendations

Switch to a piperazine phenothiazine or a nonphenothiazine.

Lesions of the Lens

Presentation

Fine white or yellow-brown granules appear in the anterior capsule. They are visible with a penlight (if granular deposits are heavy) or an ophthalmoscope. A stellate pattern of granular deposits is typical.

Incidence

The condition appears to be dose-related (cumulative), usually with high doses given for extended periods of time. Granules are usually visible after a total dose of 1000 g chlorpromazine. Incidence increases significantly above a total cumulative dose of 2500 g chlorpromazine. Lens deposits are usually seen in patients who have received more than 300 mg/day for 2 years or more. Phenothiazines, especially chlorpromazine, are more often implicated, but lesions have also been reported with thiothixene.

Mechanism

The parent drug or a metabolite interacts with protein or melanin in UV light. Neuroleptics may also affect melanocyte-inhibiting factor.

Clinical Significance

The granular deposits do not interfere with visual acuity except in advanced stages and are reversible after the drug is discontinued. In advanced stages, the patient may complain about dark or cloudy vision with poor adaptation to light changes.

Recommendations

Decrease the dose or switch to a piperazine phenothiazine or a nonphenothiazine.

Retinitis Pigmentosa

Presentation

There is dark film over the retina. Clumps of pigment are also seen. The lesion is visible with fundoscopy.

Incidence

The incidence is related to dose and duration.

Chlorpromazine-induced retinopathy is associated with high total dose (100.0 g or more) over 2 years or more. A clear relationship between chlorpromazine and retinopathy is unproven because patients were also treated with other phenothiazines, namely, thioridazine.

Thioridazine is most widely known for causing retinopathy, which is most likely to occur at doses greater than 1200 mg/day for 4–8 weeks. It has been very rarely reported in doses of less than 800 mg/day. The manufacturer argues that in many cases, patients who developed retinopathy while on thioridazine also had a history of taking other neuroleptics, primarily chlorpromazine.

Mechanism

Phenothiazines or their metabolites are absorbed by melanin, and the accumulation can lead to changes that may interfere with the pigment epithelium's ability to eliminate desquamated rod segments. There also appear to be alterations in the enzyme system of the photoreceptor cells (rods and cones) that result in the impairment of rhodopsin formation and amino acid incorporation, with eventual destruction of cells (all based on animal studies).

Clinical Significance

Patients may complain of blurring or brown discoloration of vision and difficulty seeing at night. Loss of visual acuity is usually reported before pigmentation is seen. Early identification of pigmentary changes or decreased vision together with discontinuation of the phenothiazine or lowering of the dose may prevent further damage. Pigmentation is generally considered irreversible, but may decrease, disappear, or remain unchanged after the drug is discontinued.

Recommendations

1. Discontinue thioridazine or chlorpromazine and switch to a piperazine phenothiazine or a nonphenothiazine.
2. Patients on long-term or high-dose aliphatic/piperidine phenothiazine therapy should have an ophthalmologic exam at least yearly.
3. Do not exceed the FDA-approved upper limit for thioridazine (800 mg/day) in chronic treatment.

Suggested Readings

Bond W. S., Yee G. C.: Ocular and cutaneous effects of chronic phenothiazine therapy. *Am J Hosp Pharm* 37:74–78, 1980.
Connell M. M. *et al:* Chorioretinopathy associated with thioridazine therapy. *Arch Ophthalmol* 71:816–821, 1964.
Davidorf F. H.: Thioridazine pigmentary retinopathy. *Arch Ophthalmol* 90:251–255, 1973.
Satanova A.: Pigmentation due to phenothiazines in high and prolonged dosage. *J Am Med Assoc* 191:263–268, 1965.
Shader R. I., DiMascio A.: *Psychotropic Drug Side Effects.* Baltimore, Williams & Wilkins, 1970, pp 107–115.

PREGNANCY: TERATOGENICITY

Incidence

The literature shows few data for a definite correlation between the use of psychotropics and teratogenicity. According to Neurnberg *et al*, 1984: "Controlled studies have indicated that phenothiazines can be safely administered to pregnant women without the danger of teratogenic effects and isolated reports do not provide enough evidence for incriminating phenothiazines." Many studies have been done using phenothiazines, but the same can be said for the other neuroleptics. No significant difference was found between controls and haloperidol-treated mothers with regard to teratogenic effects. However, there are two isolated cases of limb reduction after haloperidol administration (Kopelman *et al*, 1975).

Mechanism

Teratogenicity is dependent on dosage, duration of treatment, tissue distribution, state of fetal development, genetic susceptibility of the fetus, and time of administration (compared to gestation time).

The important variable that determines whether a drug will have a teratogenic effect is timing. The first trimester is a critical period when the embryo undergoes rapid organ development and shows extreme sensitivity to any medication. It is during this period of time that major malformations may be induced.

The second and third trimesters are periods of further growth and development, and although teratogenic changes can occur, the fetus shows some resistance to teratogens. Changes that can occur during this period include a reduction in cell size and number.

Recommendations

1. Caution should be observed in administering any medications during the first trimester.
2. Controlled studies have indicated that teratogenic effects with psychotropics do not occur with greater frequency as compared with controls.
3. If use of a neuroleptic is absolutely indicated, a phenothiazine (chlorpromazine) may be a good choice.

4. At present, it may not be appropriate to recommend haloperidol during the first trimester.
5. Studies with newer antipsychotics are not extensive; therefore, similar precautions should be taken.

Suggested Readings

Kopelman A. E., McCullan F. W., Heggeness L.: Limb malformations following maternal use of haloperidol. *J Am Med Assoc* 231:62–64, 1975.

Neurnberg H. G., Prudic J.: Guidelines for treatment or psychosis during pregnancy. *Hosp Community Psychiatry* 35:67–71, 1984.

RENAL EFFECTS

Presentation, Incidence, and Mechanism

Urinary retention or incontinence is more commonly seen with antipsychotics that have high anticholinergic activity; the patients primarily affected are those predisposed (e.g., the elderly). Painful urination (dysuria) is less frequently encountered. One case of retroperitoneal fibrosis has been reported with haloperidol. Acute renal failure due to rhabdomyolysis may occur following frequent intramuscular injections of neuroleptics.

Clinical Significance and Recommendations

Most urinary retention or incontinence is benign in younger patients and will remit on reduction of dosage or discontinuation of antiparkinson drugs. If symptoms are severe or persistent, a urological examination should be conducted, particularly in the elderly. Small doses of bethanecol have been advocated to reduce the peripheral manifestations of anticholinergic effects such as urinary retention. Retroperitoneal fibrosis is a very rare but serious complication that affects the kidneys and should receive immediate attention. Try to reduce frequent use of the intramuscular route to prevent complications resulting from rhabdomyolysis.

Monitoring of CPK levels and urinary myoglobin is recommended for patients who develop muscular discomfort, nausea, or confusion while receiving frequent intramuscular injections of neuroleptics.

Suggested Readings

Jeffries J. J. *et al:* Retroperitoneal fibrosis and haloperidol. *Am J Psychiatry* 139:1524–1525, 1982.
Thase M. E., Shostak M.: Rhabdomyolysis complicating rapid intramuscular neuroleptization. *J Clin Psychopharmacol* 4:46–48, 1984.

SUDDEN DEATH

Presentation

This is an ''autopsy negative'' or unexpected death in an otherwise apparently healthy person taking neuroleptic medication.

Incidence

Sudden death is extremely rare.

Mechanism

Sudden death is postulated to result from ventricular tachycardia or fibrillation, ventricular asystole or bradycardia, or sudden large decreases in cardiac output resulting from ventricular failure or vasodepressor reflexes. Since neuroleptics have arrhythmogenic potential, they have been implicated as a risk factor in sudden death. It has also been postulated that increased acid mucopolysaccharide deposits in the cardiovascular system by neuroleptics may be of etiological significance in causing sudden death. Laryngeal–pharyngeal dystonia may also be a factor in causing sudden death due to asphyxiation.

Clinical Significance

The relationship between neuroleptics and sudden death is controversial, and there are no good data at present to indicate that sudden death is more common in patients receiving neuroleptics. Sudden death occurs rarely throughout the general population and was noted to occur in psychiatric patients before the advent of neuroleptic drugs. There are also other factors that may be more important than medication, including age, sex, underlying heart disease, diabetes, hypertension, smoking, and even intense stress or emotional states. At present, it is prudent to assess the cardiovascular and respiratory status of any patient before prescribing neuroleptic medication. When employing rapid neuroleptization techniques, it would also be prudent to observe for any changes in the cardiovascular status.

Suggested Readings

Brown R. P., Kocsis J. K.: Sudden death and antipsychotic drugs. *Hosp Community Psychiatry* 35:486–491, 1984.
Ellman J. P.: Sudden death. *Can J Psychiatry* 25:331–333, 1982.
Flaherty J. A., Lahmeyer H. W.: Laryngeal–pharyngeal dystonia as a possible cause of asphyxia and haloperidol. *Am J Psychiatry* 135:1414–1415, 1978.

SYNDROME OF INAPPROPRIATE ANTIDIURETIC HORMONE

Presentation

In the reported drug-induced cases, clinical findings included lethargy, disorientation, confusion, seizures, and coma/semicomatose state. Accompanying laboratory findings included: (1) hyponatremia and hypoosmolarity of serum; (2) inappropriate large amounts of sodium in the urine despite hyponatremia; (3) absence of signs of dehydration or overhydration; (4) normal renal, adrenal, and thyroid function; and (5) urine that was less than maximally dilute when compared with plasma osmolality.

Incidence

The occurrence of the syndrome of inappropriate antidiuretic hormone (SIADH) is rare. Water intoxication or the SIADH or both have been reported with thiothixene, thioridazine, fluphenazine, haloperidol, chlorpromazine, and loxapine.

The onset occurred after a varied length of therapy on a neuroleptic. One author reported a case with the onset 4 hr after the last dose of thioridazine (500 mg total given over a period of 9 hr) Rao et al, 1975. Others report onset of symptoms after months of continuous neuroleptic therapy.

Mechanism

The exact mechanism of action is not known. In animal studies with phenothiazines, two mechanisms for phenothiazine effect on vasopressin have been proposed: (1) the existence of an alternative pathway for vasopressin release that did not involve a cholinergic step and (2) different influences on cholinergic neurons by phenothiazines. Some derivatives act as cholinomimetics, e.g., promethazine (stimulating a release of vasopressin), and others as acetycholine antagonists, e.g., chlorpromazine (inhibiting vasopressin release). Differences in the action of various phenothiazines may be related to their different molecular structures (side-chain length, branching on the side chain, and size of groups attached to the terminal nitrogen on the side chain).

Another suggested mechanism is that the SIADH may be associated with a hypothalamic involvement. Support for this hypothesis is that of the close proximity of the thirst and ADH-releasing center to the limbic area. Another possible mechanism is via direct stimulation of the hypothalamic thirst center.

Also, a mechanism similar to that hypothesized for tardive dyskinesia can be involved: (1) denervation of postsynaptic dopamine neurons and a resulting supersensitivity and (2) an increase in presynaptic neural secretion of dopamine via a feedback mechanism. The consequent effect would be an increase in thirst or ADH secretion or both, resulting in water intoxication.

Recommendations

1. Discontinue the suspected offending agent.
2. Restrict fluids and free water intake.

Therapeutic response is reported to be dramatic, consciousness being regained and lab findings being normalized within 24–96 hr.

Suggested Readings

DeRivera J. L.: Inappropriate secretion of antidiuretic hormone from fluphenazine therapy (letter). *Ann Intern Med* 82(6):811–812, 1975.

Dyball R. E.: The effects of drugs on the release of vasopressin. *Br J Pharmacol Chemother* 33:29–41, 1968.

Mutak F., Kalynaraman K.: Syndrome of inappropriate secretion of antidiuretic hormone in patients treated with psychotherapeutic drugs. *Arch Neurol* 34:374–375, 1977.

Rao K. J., Miller M., Moses A.: Water intoxication and thioridazine (letter). *Ann Intern Med* 82:61, 1975.

Raskind M. A., Orenstein H., Graham C.: Acute psychosis, increased water ingestion and inappropriate antidiuretic hormone secretion. *Am J Psychiatry* 132(9):907–910, 1975.

Smith W. O., Clark M. L.: Self-induced water intoxication in schizophrenic patients. *Am J Psychiatry* 137(9):1055–1060, 1980.

Vincent F. M., Emery S.: Antidiuretic hormone syndrome and thioridazine (letter). *Ann Intern Med* 89(1):147–148, 1978.

MISCELLANEOUS EFFECTS

Dysphagia (difficulty in swallowing): Difficulty in swallowing, leading to choking, has occasionally been associated with neuroleptics.

Moss H., Green A.: Neuroleptic-associated dysphagia confirmed by esophageal manometry. *Am J Psychiatry* 139:515–516, 1982.

Epistaxis (nosebleed): Epistaxis was reported in three hypertensive patients receiving thioridazine; it is probably an idiosyncratic reaction that can be stopped by discontinuing the drug or switching the patient to another antipsychotic agent.

Idupaganti S.: Epistaxis in hypertensive patients taking thioridazine. *Am J Psychiatry* 139:1083–1084, 1982.

Hyperglycemia: There was a case report of hyperglycemia in a 49-year-old female taking loxitane and amoxapine. The common metabolite 7-OH amoxapine was implicated. However, the patient was also taking lithium, which may have contributed to her hyperglycemia.
Tollefson G., Laser T.: Nonketotic hyperglycemia associated with loxitane and amoxapine: Case report. *J Clin Psychiatry* 44:374–378, 1983.

Neuroleptic separation anxiety syndrome: This is a new side effect that has been proposed to explain the development of school phobia in young patients treated for Tourette's syndrome with neuroleptics.
Linet L.: Tourette syndrome, pimozide, and school phobia; the neuroleptic separation anxiety syndrome. *Am J Psychiatry* 142:613–615, 1985.
The existence of this side effect has been challenged and thought to represent a facet of akathisia.
Heiser J., Sramek J.: More on Tourette syndrome and school phobia. *Am J Psychiatry* 143:265, 1986.

Nightmares: There were three cases reported in female patients of ages 27, 42, and 68 years. The dose of thiothixene was from 5 to 20 mg at bedtime. In addition to nightmares, patients reported feeling anxious, tremor, tachycardia, and in one case a feeling of smothering. A possible mechanism may include REM or Stage IV disturbances.
Solomon K.: Thiothixene and bizarre nightmares: An association. *J Clin Psychiatry* 44:77–78, 1983.

Priapism (painful penile erection): There was a case report of a 25-year-old black male treated with 30 mg/day of fluphenazine. The author proposed that antipsychotics lead to cholinergic dominance.
Fishbain D. A.: Priapism resulting from fluphenazine treatment reversed by diphenhydramine. *Ann Emerg Med* 14:600–602, 1985.

Retroperitoneal fibrosis: A case of renal fibrosis was attributed to haloperidol; the condition should be differentiated from other causes of obstructive uropathy.
Jeffries J., Lyall W., Bezchibnyk K., et al: Retroperitoneal fibrosis and haloperidol. *Am J Psychiatry* 139:1524–1525, 1982.

Rhabdomyolysis: There was a case report in a 23-year-old male; rhabdomyolysis was attributed to haloperidol, 30 mg/day PO with a genetic predisposition to rhabdomyolysis.
Cavannaugh J. J., Finalyson R. E.: Rhabdomyolysis due to acute dystonic reaction to antipsychotic drugs. *J Clin Psychiatry* 45:356–357, 1984.

Seborrheic dermatitis: Of a total of 42 patients with neuroleptic-induced parkinsonism, 25 developed seborrheic dermatitis. Psuedoparkinsonism reactions may occur in patients predisposed to this side effect. Seborrheic dermatitis occurs after longer periods of neuroleptic medication use and does not appear in acute treatment.

Binder R. L., Jonelis F. J.: Seborrheic dermatitis: A newly reported side effect of neuroleptics. *J Clin Psychiatry* 45:125–126, 1984.

Suicide attempts: There are several reports of neuroleptic-induced akathisia associated with suicides.

Drake R., Erhlich J.: Suicide attempts associated with akathisia. *Am J Psychiatry* 142:499–501, 1985.

Tardive dystonia: Tardive dystonia is a rare type of movement disorder induced by neuroleptics that is characterized by the appearance of a chronic and often painful dystonia. A review of 351 inpatients revealed that 7 (2%) suffered from this condition and that mostly young males were affected.

Yassa R., Nair V., Dimitry R.: Prevalence of tardive dystonia. *Acta Psychiatr Scand* 73:629–633, 1986.

Tics: Two 9-year-old boys with hyperactivity disorders developed tics on low doses of antipsychotics. The tics, which included movements of the face, neck, and shoulders as well as throat-clearing sounds, disappeared following withdrawal of the drugs.

Gualtieri C. T., Patterson D. R.: Neuroleptic-induced tics in two hyperactive children. *Am J Psychiatry* 143:1176–1177, 1986.

Torsade de Pointes: A 53-year-old male, treated with thioridazine, 150 mg BID, developed Torsade de Pointes, which was treated unsuccessfully with lidocaine, but responded to an IV drip of isoproterenol, 0.2 mg/min.

Kemper A. J.: Thioridazine-induced Torsade de Pointes: Successful therapy with isoproterenol. *J Am Med Assoc* 249:2931–2934, 1983.

Vein thrombosis: There were three case reports; the patients were 37, 64, and 81 years of age. The medications used were chlorpromazine and thioridazine. The authors speculate that thrombosis may be caused by phenothiazines causing an increase in platelet aggregation.

Varia I., Krishnan R. R., Davidson J.: Deep vein thrombosis with antipsychotic drugs. *Psychosomatics* 24:1097–1098, 1983.

2

Reactions to Antidepressants: Tricyclic and Tetracyclic

ANTICHOLINERGIC EFFECTS

Incidence

Anticholinergic side effects are common and annoying adverse effects.

Mechanism

Among the mechanisms of the various effects are as follows:

1. Muscarinic-receptor-blocking properties.
2. Dry mouth—salivary gland inhibition.
3. Blurred vision—due to blockade of the sphincter and ciliary muscle of the eye. This blockade results in mydriasis and paralysis of visual accommodation.
4. Urinary hesitancy and retention—increased bladder sphincter tone and volume of fluid necessary to trigger detrusor contraction.
5. Constipation and paralytic ileus—due to decreased gastrointestinal motility.

Clinical Significance

A history of previous adverse effects of similar anti-cholinergic drugs or a history of existing disease (glaucoma, benign prostatic hypertrophy, constipation) should alert the clinician to the possibility of future problems.

Anticholinergic side effects will usually appear early in treatment or with increasing dosage, with some tolerance developing during continued therapy. They may also improve with a decrease in dosage.

Preexisting narrow-angle glaucoma can be exacerbated by the anticholinergic effects, unless it is already managed with medication. An antidepressant with low anticholinergic side effects (e.g., nortriptyline, desipramine) may be more preferable in a patient with the narrow-angle type.

Presentation and Recommendations

Gastrointestinal: Dry mouth can lead to a bad taste in the mouth and difficulty in speaking. The condition is easily alleviated by having the patient suck on sugarless candy (sugar and dry mouth may make the patient more susceptible to dental caries) or use artificial saliva.

Constipation: This is more likely to occur with an increased intake of bulk foods and decreased fluid intake. Mild laxatives, i.e., bulk-producing stool softners, should be used before the more potent laxatives, i.e., saline, irritant/stimulant laxatives, are initiated. More serious situations such as paralytic ileus can arise and can be potentially life-threatening, especially in the elderly.

Genitourinary: Urinary hesitancy and retention can become a serious problem, especially in males with prostatic hypertrophy. Cholinergic agents, e.g., bethanecol, have been used to reverse the muscarinic blockade.

Ophthalmic: Near vision is usually blurred and distant vision is left intact. The blurring may lessen with continued duration of treatment.

Central anticholinergic syndrome: This is usually due to a large dose of a drug with strong anticholinergic effects or to the combined effect of several drugs. Elderly patients may be more susceptible. Clinically, the syndrome appears as an acute toxic confusional psychosis. Symptoms include hallucinations, bizzare motor behavior, disorientation, confusion, delirium, anxiety, and hyperactivity. There are peripheral anticholinergic symptoms accompanying central toxic signs: tachycardia, mydriasis, increased temperature, flushed face, decreased bowel sounds, urinary retention, warm, dry skin, and increased respiratory rate. Treatment includes discontinuation of the drug and supportive treatment. Physostigmine has been used, but has limited use due to its short half-life. Phenothiazine neuroleptics with high anticholinergic activity, particularly thioridazine and chlorpromazine, should not be used to treat the psychotic symptoms, because they can exacerbate the anticholinergic toxicity.

Suggested Readings

Blackwell B.: Adverse effects of antidepressant drugs. Part I. *Drugs* 21:201–219, 1981.

Everett H. C.: The use of bethanecol chloride with tricyclic antidepressants. *Am J Psychiatry* 132(11):1202–1204, 1975.

Johnson A. L., Hollister L. E., Berger P. A.: The anticholinergic intoxication syndrome: Diagnosis and treatment. *J Clin Psychiatry* 42:313–317, 1981.

Hvidos A. J., Bennett J. A., Wells B. G., *et al:* Anticholinergic psychosis in a patient receiving usual doses of haloperidol, desipramine and benztropine. *Clin Pharm* 2:174–178, 1983.

BLOOD DYSCRASIAS

Presentation

Agranulocytosis: The average latency is 4–8 weeks after medication is initiated. The clinical presentation may include fever, pharyngitis, dysphagia, stomatitis, lymphadenopathy, or other signs of infection (e.g., mucosal ulcers).

Incidence

Agranulocytosis: This reaction is rare. Elderly patients may be more prone. The condition may be more prevalent in females. Cases have been reported with imipramine, amitriptyline, and amoxapine.

Thrombocytopenia purpura: There are isolated case reports with doxepin, amitriptyline, imipramine, and desipramine.

Mechanism

Agranulocytosis: The suggested mechanisms include: (1) allergic reaction and (2) direct toxic effect of the drug or its metabolite on granulocyte precursors.

Thrombocytopenic purpura: The suggested mechanism is an allergic hypersensitivity reaction.

Clinical Significance

In case reports of hematological reactions, the antidepressant was often not the only drug being prescribed when the reaction developed.

Cross-tolerance among tricyclics has not been established; therefore, a safer treatment alternative may be with a structurally unrelated agent.

In patients with leukopenia, you can often continue safely with medication. In some cases, the WBC returned to normal *with* continued therapy with the suspected agent, which raises the question whether the occurrence of leukopenia was unrelated to drug therapy. Leukopenia does not automatically lead to the development of agranulocytosis.

In general, routine screening of white blood cells would be of little value due to the low incidence of blood dyscrasias. If you receive *one* abnormal WBC value, repeat the WBC before deeming this first low value significant. Baseline blood work before initiation of medication is recommended. If symptoms or complaints of infection are present, then a thorough blood work-up would be warranted.

Recommendations

Agranulocytosis:

1. Discontinue the drug immediately.
2. Guard against or treat any infection.

Suggested Readings

Albertini K. S., Penders T. M.: Agranulocytosis associated with tricyclics. *J Clin Psychiatry* 39:483–485, 1978.
Blackwell B.: Adverse effects of antidepressant drugs. *Drugs* 21(3):201–219, 1981.
Christenson B. C.: Agranulocytosis associated with amoxapine. *Am J Psychiatry* 140(7):921–922, 1983.
Litvak R., Kaelbling R.: Agranulocytosis, leukopenia and psychotropic drugs. *Arch Gen Psychiatry* 24:266–267, 1971.

CARDIOVASCULAR EFFECTS

Conduction Delays

Presentation

Electrocardiographic (ECG) changes include prolonged PR, QRS, and QT intervals, and flattened or inverted T waves, and resemble the effects produced by quinidine and procainamide. There are also direct effects on the heart, including an anticholinergic effect, which may lead to sinus tachycardia (increased heart rate). Conduction effects (ECG changes) may interact with anticholinergic effects to produce arrhythmias or heart block.

Incidence

Of the tricyclics, tertiary amines produce the most pronounced conduction effects, followed by doxepin and the secondary amine tricyclics (nortriptyline and desipramine). ECG changes with maprotiline are similar to those with the tricyclics. Amoxapine can produce some ECG changes sim-

ilar to those produced by the tricyclics, but the incidence
appears to be lower. Trazodone appears devoid of conduction
or inotropic effects at therapeutic doses. With most antidepressants, however, the incidence of clinically serious ECG
changes is very low, except in overdose.

Mechanism

Tricyclic antidepressants prolong conduction time
through the bundle of His, the right and left bundle branches,
and the Purkinje fibers; these effects are similar to those
produced by quinidine. Tricyclics also have a negative inotropic effect (weakened contractility). Trazodone seems to
produce no slowing of conduction times.

Clinical Significance

In normal, healthy patients, these conduction changes
are not cause for concern when usual doses of these drugs are
prescribed. However, in patients with preexisting cardiac
disease, tricyclic and tetracyclic compounds may induce
PVCs, or supraventricular or ventricular tachycardias or both.
Some experts have postulated that these arrhythmias may be
the mechanism for rare occurrences of sudden death with
tricyclic compounds.

A small increase in heart rate (tachycardia) due to an
anticholinergic effect is common with most antidepressants
and is rarely cause for concern.

Recommendations

The possibility of conduction changes should not lead to
withholding antidepressant medication from most depressed
cardiac patients, except in those with severe cardiac disease
(i.e., heart block or post-myocardial infarction), in whom the
possibility of inducing added conduction defects is contraindicated. In selecting an antidepressant, one must also consider
the hazards of orthostatic hypotension and tachycardia. Base-
line and follow-up ECG monitoring will be essential in

patients who are at risk from conduction changes. Trazodone may be safer than conventional tricyclics in patients with conduction defects. When in doubt, or with elderly patients, a base-line ECG will identify those patients for whom even slight conduction changes would not be desirable. Antidepressant overdose (as little as one week's supply) is an acute medical emergency, often requiring intensive cardiac monitoring and treatment of life-threatening arrhythmias and ECG changes.

There are several reports of heart block with trazodone; although such block is perhaps rare, there is still need for caution when prescribing this drug for high-risk patients.

Suggested Readings

Himmelhoch J. M.: Cardiovascular effects of trazodone. *J Clin Psychopharmacol* 1(6)Suppl:76–81, 1981.

Rausch J. L., Pavlinac D. M., Newman P. E.: Complete heart block following a single dose of trazodone. *Am J Psychiatry* 141:1472–1473, 1984.

Rosenfeld L. E., Langou R. E.: Cardiovascular effects of tricyclic antidepressants: A brief review. *Hosp Formulary* 1981:604–608, 1981.

Orthostatic Hypotension

Presentation

An abnormal orthostatic drop in blood pressure is often defined as 15 mm Hg diastolic or greater. Watch for associated subjective complaints such as dizziness or lightheadedness.

Incidence

The incidence is about 20% in patients receiving therapeutic doses of imipramine (100–400 mg daily); the reaction is more likely to occur in elderly patients receiving imipramine or amitriptyline, less commonly with secondary amine tricyclics. The incidence with newer, "second generation'' antidepressants is similar or may be less than that with tricyclics.

Mechanism

Orthostatic hypotension has been attributed to the central blockade of α-adrenergic receptors, a peripheral antiadrenergic effect, and a myocardial depressant effect; the exact mechanism remains uncertain.

Clinical Significance

There is increased risk of falls, particularly in the elderly or in those with preexisting cardiovascular disease.

Recommendations

Check blood pressure for postural changes (e.g., sitting and standing BP) before prescribing antidepressants for high-risk patients. If possible, use drugs that are less likely to induce postural changes; caution patients not to rise too quickly from sedentary positions. Although there is no tolerance to this effect with time, starting with smaller doses and increasing slowly will help the patient cope better with any postural effects. In the elderly, it might be advisable to avoid large single bedtime dosing and thus reduce the risk of falls and fractures. Profound hypotension, such as that associated with antidepressant overdose, is a medical emergency.

Suggested Readings

Cassem N.: Cardiovascular effects of antidepressants. *J Clin Psychiatry* 43:11(Sect 2):22–29, 1982.
Roose S. P., Glassman A. H., Siris S. G., *et al:* Comparison of imipramine and nortriptyline-induced orthostatic hypotension: A meaningful difference. *J Clin Psychopharmacol* 1(5):316–319, 1981.

DERMATOLOGICAL EFFECTS

Presentation

Skin reactions reported include urticaria, photosensitivity, and cutaneous vasculitis. Urticarial reactions are the most commonly seen.

Incidence

Since rashes are common in general, it is difficult to determine whether the suspected drug is the actual cause.

Maprotilene has an increased incidence of skin rashes as compared to other antidepressants—an overall incidence of 3% after 2 weeks of treatment. Reports of an allergic reaction are slightly higher with amitriptyline than with imipramine.

Mechanism

The reaction is probably of an allergic type.

Clinical Significance

If a drug is discontinued due to a possible skin reaction, and the reaction subsequently clears up, it may be necessary to rechallenge the patient to determine a valid cause-and-effect relationship.

Recommendations

1. Discontinuation of the suspected drug is not always necessary, since the rash may clear despite continued treatment.
2. When the suspected drug is discontinued, the rash will usually clear in a few days.
3. For symptomatic relief for the rash, a mild topical steroid or antihistamine or both can be used for a short term.

Suggested Readings

Blackwell, B.: Adverse effects of antidepressant drugs. Part I. *Drugs* 21(3):201–219, 1981.

Blackwell B.: Adverse effects of antidepressant drugs. Part 2. *Drugs* 21(4):273–282, 1981.

Litvak R., Kaelbling R.: Dermatological side effects with psychotropics. *Dis Nerv Sys* 33:309–311, 1972.

Pinder R. M. *et al:* Maprotilene: A review of its pharmacological properties and therapeutic efficacy in mental depressive states. *Drugs* 13(5):321–352, 1977.

ENDOCRINE EFFECTS

Galactorrhea and Amenorrhea

Presentation

The patient may complain of increased swelling and tenderness of the breast, as well as lactation.

Incidence

Although listed in the package insert of most antidepressants, these reactions are very rarely reported in the world literature. There are four cases of galactorrhea noted in the literature, two of which were associated with amoxapine, one with imipramine, and one with amitriptyline. Of the two cases with amoxapine, one also included amenorrhea.

Mechanism

Galactorrhea and amenorrhea are generally an adverse effect of antipsychotics. This reaction is attributed to elevated levels of prolactin brought about by blockage of the dopamine receptors in the tubuloinfundibular part of the brain. Except for amoxapine, most antidepressants have negligible dopamine-blocking effects.

Clinical Significance

Amenorrhea may be falsely interpreted by the patient as pregnancy.

Recommendations

If there is a history of irregular periods or problems of galactorrhea, it may be wise to avoid amoxapine. However, the number of cases of galactorrhea and amenorrhea reported is extremely small.

Suggested Readings

Galenberg, A. J., Cooper D. S., Doller J. C., *et al:* Galactorrhea and hyperprolactinemia associated with amoxapine therapy. *J Am Med Assoc* 242(17):1900–1902, 1979.

Jaffe K., Zisook S.: Galactorrhea in a patient treated with amoxapine. *J Clin Psychiatry* 39:821, 1978.

Klein J. J., Segal R. L., Warner R. R.: Galactorrhea due to imipramine. *N Engl J Med* 271:510–512, 1964.

Rees, W. D.: Lactation and ovarian cyst formation following treatment with amitriptyline. *Practitioner* 198:835–838, 1967.

Sexual Dysfunction

Presentation

Sexual dysfunctions may surface as the patient's depressive symptomatology improves because of a greater frequency of sexual activity. Therefore, sexual problems may occur after 1–2 months of therapy, except for priapism with trazodone, which may occur after only 1–2 weeks of therapy. The major dysfunctions covered in the literature include problems with erectile dysfunction, changes in the quality of orgasm, ejaculatory dysfunctions, and priapism. Unfortunately, the literature deals mostly with sexual problems in the male, with little information on the female, partly because the male response is more visible and quantifiable. For

example, painful intercourse for the female may be the result
of an antidepressant with high anticholinergic properties decreasing vaginal lubrication.

Incidence

Available information consists of individual case reports
or a small series of cases for each medication. The number of
cases for each medication may reflect varying thoroughness
of pharmaceutical companies in monitoring these problems
and may not indicate the relative risk. The new generation
antidepressants seem to have a lower incidence of sexual side
effects. The one notable exception is trazodone, which has
been associated with priapism (sustained penile erection,
usually unaccompanied by sexual desire and often painful) in
the male and also reports of clitoral tumescence in the
female. The association between priapism and trazodone has
been reported in 21 cases, with 7 patients needing surgical
intervention as of January 1983; more than 100 cases were
reported by 1986. In addition, three case reports of increased
libido associated with trazodone in women have been noted
(see the Miscellaneous Effects section at the end of the
chapter).

Mechanism

Sexual dysfunctions are the results of imbalances in
autonomic and central nervous system mechanisms in the
nervous system. It is proposed that the parasympathetic and
sympathetic nervous systems are responsible for autonomic
changes, and elevated prolactin levels are associated with
central mechanisms. These effects are similar to the action of
neuroleptics, with less activity on prolactin levels. The possible exception is amoxapine, which does alter prolactin levels.
Medications with high anticholinergic properties are associated with erectile disturbance, and medications associated
with effects on the sympathetic nervous system may cause
ejaculatory problems. Since these medications affect two or
three physiological systems, it is important to remember that

more than one type of sexual dysfunction may occur. Reviews conclude that most antidepressants affect orgasm and ejaculation, but, with the exception of trazodone, have a minor effect on erection.

Clinical Significance

The clinician, because of his own anxiety, may fail to ask the patient questions in this area, leading to noncompliance with the medication regimen. In addition, because of our lack of understanding of sexual dysfunction in depressive illnesses, sexual dysfunction may be erroneously attributed to the illness.

Recommendations

1. Rule out medical conditions that may cause sexual impairment.
2. Before starting antidepressant therapy, evaluate sexual activity.
3. If a sexual problem presents after 1–2 months of therapy, consider another antidepressant.
4. Bear in mind that depressive illnesses are frequently associated with sexual dysfunction.
5. Cyproheptadine, 4 mg (2 hr before attempting sexual stimulation), may be prescribed for females who are experiencing anorgasmia caused by serotonergic antidepressants.
6. If priapism with trazodone is not responsive to drug discontinuation, consider metaraminol (injected directly into cavernous of the penis). Priapism is a medical emergency; left untreated the patient may permanently experience erectile dysfunction.

Suggested Readings

Communication concerning trazodone: Mead Johnson Pharmaceutical Division (812) 428–5128.

Diego D., Magni G.: Sexual side effects of antidepressant drugs. *Psychosomatics* 24:1076–1081, 1983.

Harrison W. M., Rabkin J. G., Ehrhart A. A., et al: Effects of antidepressant medication on sexual function: A controlled study. *J Clin Psychopharmacol* 6(3):144–149, 1986.

Kowalski A., Dinnerstein S. L., Burrows G., et al: The sexual side-effects of antidepressant medication: A double-blind comparison of two antidepressants in a non-psychiatric population. *Br J Psychiatry* 147:413–418, 1985.

Mitchell J. E., Popkin M. K.: Antidepressant drug therapy and sexual dysfunction in men: A review. *J Clin Psychopharmacol* 3(2):76–79, 1983.

Scher M., Krieger J. N., Juergen S.: Trazodone and priapism. *Am J Psychiatry* 140(10):1362–1363, 1983.

Steele T. E., Howell E. F.: Cyproheptadine for imipramine-induced anorgasmia. *J Clin Psychopharmacol* 6(5):326–327, 1986.

Weight Gain

Presentation

The patient may gain 10 pounds or more over a 2-month period. Generally, this gain does not lead to obesity. There has been peripheral edema associated with up to 11-pound weight gains in patients treated with trazodone; however, the weight gain occurred in 6–8 days of therapy and decreased with dosage reduction. The mechanism of causing weight gain with Trazodone appears to differ from that of other antidepressants.

Incidence

The incidence of weight gain is difficult to ascertain because there have been mainly case reports and few studies. Although the incidence has not been reported, the occurrence of weight and appetite changes has been noted by clinician and patient. The phenomenon is difficult to study, because of the multitude of other variables.

Mechanism

The postulated mechanisms for weight gain have included the following: (1) A central mechanism in the hypothalamus may be responsible for an increased need for calories; (2) people with depression begin to increase their caloric intake; (3) the sedative effects of antidepressants may decrease activity and contribute to weight gain; (4) histamine-receptor blockade may play a role in appetite-stimulating effects (Table 1) and drug-induced changes in carbohydrate metabolism.

Clinical Significance

The importance of maintaining an adequate diet cannot be overemphasized. However, an abnormal gain in weight may occur and reduce compliance or cause the patient to stop taking the medication. In patients with weight gain, concerns should be assessed more frequently. A past history of appetite and weight gain may be a significant factor in weight gain.

Recommendations

1. Use a medication with the least amount of anti-histamine effect (e.g., desipramine) in patients who are obese or have a past history of weight problems.
2. Have the patient exercise every other day (also beneficial for depression).
3. Make a diary of caloric intake if weight gain appears.
4. A history of weight changes should be noted during the initial evaluation.

Table 1. Antihistamine Potency

Doxepine	HIGH	
Amitriptyline	↑	Increasing antihistamine effect
Imipramine		
Nortriptyline		
Protriptyline		
Desipramine	LOW	

Suggested Readings

Barrnett J., Frances A., Kocsis J., *et al:* Peripheral edema associated with trazodone: A report of ten cases. *J Clin Psychopharmacol* 5(3):161–164, 1985.

Harris B., Young J., Hughes B.: Changes occurring in appetite and weight during short-term antidepressant treatment. *Br J Psychiatry* 145:645–648, 1984.

Paykel E. S., Mueller P. S.: Amitriptyline, weight gain and carbohydrate craving: A side effect. *Br J Psychiatry* 123:501–507, 1973.

Richelson E.: Tricyclic antidepressant and neurotransmitter receptors. *Psychiatr Ann* 9(4):186–194, 1979.

HEPATIC EFFECTS

Presentation

A variety of hepatic effects have been reported:

1. Jaundice (imipramine, desipramine, amitriptyline), usually with intrahepatic cholestasis.
2. Hepatitis (amitriptyline, imipramine).
3. Hepatic necrosis (imipramine, desipramine, amitriptyline).
4. Increased liver function tests—especially alkaline phosphatase and transaminase.

Jaundice usually presents with fever, myalgia, nausea, and anorexia for a few days preceding the appearance of bilirubinuria, jaundice, and pruritis. After the offending agent is discontinued, the symptoms usually resolve within several days to several weeks. Drug-induced chronic cholestasis is differentiated from primary biliary cirrhosis by its acute onset and tendency to resolve after discontinuation of medication. There are also certain histological features in primary biliary cirrhosis that do not appear in drug-induced cases.

Incidence

The majority of cases of hepatoxicity occur after at least 3–4 weeks of drug therapy, often at usual doses. The majority of reports have been with amitriptyline, imipramine, and desipramine. Isolated reports with other antidepressants are found in the literature. The overall incidence of hepatic abnormalities is very low (<1% with imipramine).

Mechanism

No specific mechanism is known. It is most probably a hypersensitivity reaction; some reports suggest a direct toxic effect.

Clinical Significance

Minor changes in liver function tests may occur frequently, but they are usually not significant unless there are also clinical signs of toxicity. Major changes in liver function tests should prompt an immediate medication work-up and discontinuation of the suspected drug(s).

Recommendation

1. Discontinuation of offending agents.
2. It is not necessary to perform routine liver function tests throughout antidepressant therapy. Slight increases in transaminases and alkalaine phosphatases within the high normal ranges have been noted with no clinical effect.

Suggested Readings

Herst D. A., Grace N. O., Le Compte P. M.: Prolonged cholestasis and progressive heptic fibrosis following imipramine therapy. *Gastroenterology* 79:550–554, 1980.

Maldawsky R. J.: Hepatotoxicity associated with maprotile therapy: Case report. *J Clin Psychiatry* 45:178–179, 1984.

Blackwell B.: Adverse effects of antidepressant drugs. 21(3):201–219, 1981.

NEUROLOGICAL EFFECTS

Agitation and Insomnia

Presentation

The patient experiences a sudden increase in anxiety, agitation, motor restlessness, and insomnia. These symptoms usually last for a few hours after administration of the tricyclic antidepressant.

Note: Nomifensine has amphetaminelike stimulating effects in some patients and also causes an increased incidence of insomnia. It has been withdrawn from the United States market due to serious adverse reactions (hemolytic anemia).

Incidence

These phenomena are usually observed in patients with panic attacks or when the dose of tricyclic antidepressants is started too high or increased too rapidly. Insomnia appears to be more prevalent in elderly patients.

Mechanism

The stimulatory effects of tricyclic antidepressants may result from alteration of the neurotransmitter activities in the central nervous system (CNS).

Clinical Significance

The antidepressants that possess potent stimulatory effects may be useful in treating the "retarded" type of depression.

Recommendations

1. Discontinue the tricyclic antidepressant.
2. Start the drug at a lower dose and increase the dose gradually.

3. Benzodiazepines, e.g., diazepam, can be used as an effective antidote in patients with panic attacks.
4. Substitute the present tricyclic antidepressant with a more sedative one.
5. Administer nomifensine in the morning and early afternoon, i.e., before 4:00 P.M.

Note: Nomifensine has been withdrawn from the United States market due to serious adverse reactions (hemolytic anemia).

Suggested Readings

Klein D. G., Gittleman R., Quitkin F., Rifkin A.: *Diagnosis and Drug Treatment of Psychiatric Disorders: Adults and Children,* 2nd ed. Baltimore, Williams & Wilkins, 1980, pp 449–492.
Lopez-Ibor Alino J. J., Gutierez J. L., Montejo M. L., *et al:* A double-blind clinical comparison between nomifensine and amitriptyline in the treatment of endogenous depressions. *Int Pharmacopsychiatry* 17(Suppl 1):97–105, 1982.

Central Nervous System Stimulation (Hypomania and Mania)

Presentation

Behavioral changes consist of agitation, sleeplessness, irritability, euphoria, hyperactivity, talkativeness, intrusiveness, and other manic symptoms.

Manic episodes can occur in two ways: (1) suddenly as a switch into mania during the early stage of the tricyclic treatment or (2) slowly during the maintenance treatment period.

Incidence

In patients with bipolar affective disorder, the incidence is about 30%; in patients with unipolar affective disorder, about 10%. Females are at higher risk than males.

Mechanism

The mechanism is changes in neurotransmitter, e.g., norepinephrine, serotonin, dopamine, availability and receptor sensitivity in the CNS in susceptible persons.

Clinical Significance

The "switch process" is more common in patients with a past history of manic episodes than in patients without such a past history. Patients with a history of rapid cycling respond less favorably to tricyclic antidepressants in combination with lithium than to lithium alone.

Recommendations

Discontinue tricyclic antidepressants when manic symptoms are present. Lithium salts do not alleviate the tricyclic-induced manic episodes and rapid cycling when patients are still receiving tricyclic antidepressants.

For bipolar patients, long-term maintenance tricyclic antidepressant treatments alone should be avoided, and even the combined treatment of tricyclics and lithium may not abolish the risk of cycling.

Suggested Readings

Bunney W. E.: Psychopharmacology of the switch process in affective disorders, in Lipton M. A., DiMascio A., Killam K. F. (eds): *Psychopharmacology: A Generation of Progress*. New York, Raven Press, 1978, pp 1249–1259.

Goodwin F. K.: Mood cycles as a complication in antidepressant use in affective illness. *Fair Oak Hosp Psychiatr Lett* 1:1, 1983.

Wehr T. A., Goodwin F. K.: Rapid cycling in manic depressives induced by tricyclic antidepressants. *Arch Gen Psychiatry* 36:555–559, 1979.

Zis, A. P., Goodwin F. K.: Major affective disorder as a recurrent illness. *Arch Gen Psychiatry* 36:835–839, 1979.

Electroencephalographic Changes

Tricyclic antidepressants usually cause an increase of slow waves, a decrease of alpha activity, and an increase of fast waves. More stimulating tricyclic antidepressants such as imipramine, nortriptyline, and desipramine produce fewer slow waves and more fast waves than less stimulatory tricyclic antidepressants such as amitriptyline.

After chronic multiple oral doses of amitriptyline, the electroencephalogram (EEG) was similar to that of a single dose except that a decrease in fast waves was also observed.

Protriptyline in low dosages produced changes similar to those observed in imipramine administration, but in higher dosages showed similarity to CNS stimulants (i.e., a decrease of slow waves, an increase of alpha activity, and a decrease of beta activity).

These EEG changes are considered to be of little clinical importance unless the tricyclic antidepressants are administered to patients known to have a seizure disorder. In epileptic patients, less sedative tricyclic antidepressants should be prescribed. Also, sudden dose changes and large doses should be avoided. Further titration of the daily dosage of the anticonvulsant in most cases is an adequate prophylactic measure.

Suggested Readings

Itil T. M.: The discovery of antidepressant drugs by computer-analyzed human cerebral bio-electrical potentials (CEEG). *Prog Neurol* 20:185–249, 1983.

Itil T. M., Soldatos C.: Clinical neurophysiological properties of antidepressants. *Handb Exp Pharmacol* 55(1):427–469, 1980.

Kiloh L. G., Davison K., Osselton J. W.: An electroencephalographic study of the analeptic effects of imipramine. *Electroencephalogr Clin Neurophysiol* 13:216–223, 1961.

Extrapyramidal Symptoms

1. Three patients who developed an akathisialike syndrome after the abrupt withdrawal of imipramine were reported. A link between this syndrome and dopamine turnover in the CNS was postulated. Gradual reduction of doses should prevent such syndromes.

2. Two cases of dyskinesia similar to neuroleptic-induced tardive dyskinesia were reported and attributed to the anticholinergic action from long-term exposure to tricyclic antidepressant. The dyskinetic movements should be reversible after discontinuation of the drug.

3. Nomifensine has a potent dopaminergic action that has been associated with one case of dyskinetic movements. In addition, because of other reactions, it has been removed from the United States market.

4. Amoxapine is a metabolite of loxapine that blocks postsynaptic dopaminergic receptors in the CNS. Amoxapine treatment is associated with dystonia, akathisia, parkinsonism, choreiform movements, neuroleptic malignant syndrome, and tardive dyskinesia. Affective disorders have been considered to be a possible risk factor in tardive dyskinesia: the administration of amoxapine to such patients, particularly to older women, and the long-term maintenance treatment of depression with amoxapine should be avoided unless the risk of tardive dyskinesia is justified for the patient. Usage of antiparkinsonian agents may alleviate certain types of extrapyramidal symptoms (e.g., stiffness or tremor or both).

Suggested Readings

Coccaro E. F., Siever L. J.: Second generation antidepressants: A comparative review. *J Clin Pharmacol* 25:241–260, 1985.

Fann W., Sullivan J. L., Richman B.: Dyskinesia associated with tricyclic antidepressants. *Br J Psychiatry* 128:490–493, 1976.

Gibson A. C.: Nomifensine and dyskinesia. *Br J Psychiatry* 138–439, 1981.

Satahanthan G. L., Gershon S.: Imipramine withdrawal: An akathisia-like syndrome. *Am J Psychiatry* 130:1286–1287, 1973.

Seizure Threshold

Presentation

EEG abnormalities can occur without clinical presentation of a seizure. EEG changes are more likely to be seen early after initiation of treatment, a sudden dose change, or abrupt withdrawal.

The majority of seizures are described as generalized tonic–clonic. Onset has ranged from a few days after initiation of the drug (or on increasing the dose) to weeks after initiation (or increase in dosage).

Incidence

Seizure is an uncommon phenomenon, more often associated with very large doses (or overdose) or in patients with existing seizure disorder or apparent brain damage, but can also be seen at therapeutic doses. The exact incidence is not clearly known. Figures have ranged from less than 1 to 3–4%, or as high as 15% for maprotilene. All antidepressants may lower the seizure threshold, but not to the same degree.

It has been suggested that the more sedative tricyclics (e.g., amitriptyline, imipramine, doxepine) are more epileptogenic. Maprotilene has been noted to cause grand mal seizures at therapeutic doses as well as in overdose. Although some sources indicate this as a rare occurrence, with a low incidence, other sources report a higher incidence.

Mechanism

One suggested mechanism may be related to the ability of tricyclics to block the reuptake of various brain monoamines, but the specific monoamine involved has not yet been determined.

Clinical Significance

An epileptogenic effect depends on both drug and patient factors: CNS-depressant effect of the drug, drug dosage, concomitant drug therapy (polypharmacy), sudden dosage change, preexisting EEG abnormalities, or clinical pathology.

Patients *without* a history of a seizure disorder or organicity, and with a normal EEG, are likely at low risk. In patients with existing seizure disorder or EEG abnormalities, avoidance of highly epileptogenic drugs is advised if possible.

Recommendations

In patients for whom caution should be exercised:

1. Avoid drugs with high epileptogenic properties.
2. Slowly titrate dosages.
3. Adjust the anticonvulsant medication if necessary; assess anticonvulsant levels before and after initiation of an antidepressant.
4. Weigh risk vs. benefit of drug treatment.
5. Avoid polypharmacy with multiple drugs known to affect the seizure threshold.

Discontinue the offending agent if seizures continue.

If an isolated seizure occurs in a patient with no known history of seizures, the offending agent should be discontinued and another agent used. Before prophylactic anticonvulsant therapy is considered, the patient should have a complete medical and neurological examination.

Suggested Readings

Blackwell B.: Adverse effects of antidepressant drugs. Part 1. *Drugs* 21(3):210–219, 1981.

Blackwell B.: Adverse effects of antidepressant drugs. Part 2. *Drugs* 21(4):273–282, 1981.

Giannini A. J., Price W. A.: Amoxapine-induced seizures: Case reports. *J Clin Psychiatry* 45:358–359, 1984.

Itil T. M., Soldatos C.: Epileptogenic side effects of psychotropic drugs. *J Am Med Assoc* 244(13):1460–1463, 1980.

Jabbari B., Bryan G. E., Marsh E. E., *et al:* Incidence of seizures with tricyclic and tetracyclic antidepressants. *Arch Neurol* 42:480–481, 1985.

Kim W. Y.: Seizures associated with maprotilene (letter). *Am J Psychiatry* 139(6):845–846, 1982.

Koval G., Van Nuis C., Davis T. D.: Seizures associated with amoxapine (letter). *Am J Psychiatry* 139(6):845, 1982.

Lefkowitz D., Kilgo G., Lee S.: Seizures and trazodone therapy. *Arch Gen Psychiatry* 42:523, 1985.

Remick R. A., Fine S. H.: Antipsychotic drugs and seizures. *J Clin Psychiatry* 40:78–80, 1979.

Toone B. K., Fenton G. W.: Epileptic seizures induced by psychotropic drugs. *Psychol Med* 7:265–270, 1977.

Trimble M. R.: Non-monoamine oxidase inhibitor antidepressants and epilepsy: A review. *Epilepsia* 19:241–250, 1978.

Trimble M. R.: New antidepressant drugs and the seizure threshold. *Neuropharmacology* 19:1227–1228, 1980.

Trimble M. R.: Antidepressant drugs and the seizure threshold, in Dam M., Gram L., Penry I. K. (eds): *Advances in Epileptology: 12th Epilepsy International Symposium.* New York, Raven Press, 1981.

TERATOGENIC EFFECTS

Incidence

There are only a few case reports of limb-reduction deformities attributable to tricyclic antidepressants. Two large-scale surveys have failed to implicate tricyclics in producing teratogenic effects. Several instances of apparent association between birth defects and tricyclics have been subsequently criticized because of poor or unsubstantiated temporal relationships or because the mother also ingested other drugs during the pregnancy.

Recommendations

While it is best to avoid taking any drug during pregnancy (and in particular during the first trimester), some experts feel that tricyclics may be relatively safe for use in pregnant patients when treatment is clearly indicated and there are no alternative treatments. If an antidepressant is deemed necessary, it might be best to avoid the newer "second generation" drugs, since there is little or no information available on their safety in pregnancy.

Suggested Readings

Crombi D. L., Pinsent R. J., Fleming D.: Imipramine in pregnancy. *Br Med J* 1:745, 1972.

Csernansky J. G., Hollister L. E.: Psychotropic medications: The risk of teratogenesis. *Hosp Formulary* 19:717–723, 1984.

WITHDRAWAL SYNDROMES

Presentation

The presentation of anticholinergic withdrawal may include any of the following signs and symptoms: gastrointestinal distress (nausea, vomiting, abdominal pain, diarrhea), insomnia, drowsiness, behavioral changes such as irritability, increased anxiety and agitation, apathy, withdrawal from social situations, headaches, moodiness, and worsening of underlying depression. From this extensive list, Dilsaver *et al* (1983) defined four general categories of withdrawal symptoms: (1) gastrointestinal, with or without anxiety; (2) sleep disturbance; (3) movement disorders; and (4) paradoxical activation. Most of these symptoms usually occur 1–2 days after drug discontinuation.

Incidence

The literature contains approximately 108 case reports describing the subjective and objective signs and symptoms of antidepressant withdrawal. Retrospective reviews indicate that imipramine and amitriptyine may have a 50–80% incidence of withdrawal symptoms. However, the sample sizes have been quite small and the method of detection has not been standardized.

Mechanism

Anticholinergic withdrawal leading to cholinergic rebound is the main mechanism postulated. This hypothesis may lend support to the view that antidepressants with strong anticholinergic effects are implicated more frequently in causing more severe withdrawal symptoms. Noradrenergic activation and dopaminergic activation are also considered to be associated with antidepressant withdrawal. The noradrenergic hypothesis is based on increased levels of 3-methoxy-4-hydroxyphenyl glycol (a metabolite of norepinephrine) and accompanying behavioral effects such as increased anxiety. Hyperdopaminergic states may also be implicated in withdrawal and be associated with movement disorders.

Clinical Significance

The patient may feel that his underlying depression has not improved because of erroneous attribution of withdrawal symptoms to depression. The abrupt discontinuation of medication may also exacerbate underlying medical problems.

Recommendations

1. Reinstitute antidepressant therapy and then gradually taper the drug. If withdrawal symptoms occur, a more gradual decrease is necessary.
2. If the patient develops an allergy to the medication, consider another antidepressant with a similar side effect profile.
3. In a situation of severe, abrupt withdrawal, the addition of anticholinergics may be necessary (benzotropine 1–2 mg QD or PRN).

Suggested Readings

Charney D. S., Heninger G. R., Sternberg D. E.: Abrupt discontinuation of tricyclic antidepressant drugs: Evidence for noradrenergic hyperactivity. *Br J Psychiatry* 141:377–386, 1982.

Dilsaver S. C., Greden J. F.: Antidepressant withdrawal phenomena. *Biol Psychiatry* 19(2):237–256, 1984.

Dilsaver S. C., Feinberg M., Gerden J. F.: Antidepressant withdrawal symptoms treated with anticholinergic agents. *Am J Psychiatry* 140(2):249–251, 1983.

Dilsaver S. C., Kronfol Z., Sackellares J. C., Greden J. F.: Antidepressant withdrawal syndromes: Evidence supporting the cholinergic overdrive hypothesis. *J Clin Psychopharmacol* 3(3):157–163, 1983.

Mirin S. M., Schatzberg A. F., Creasey D. E.: Mania after tricyclic antidepressant withdrawal. *Am J Psychiatry* 138:87, 1981.

Weller R. A., McKelly W. V.: Case report of withdrawal dyskinesia associated with amoxapine. *Am J Psychiatry* 140:1515, 1983.

WORSENING SCHIZOPHRENIC CONDITIONS

Presentation

The reports described either an exacerbation of preexisting schizophrenic symptomatology or a more general disor-

ganization of behavior with marked irritability and
aggressiveness.

Incidence

This effect is not noted consistently, and its occurrence
is not yet clearly defined.

Mechanism

The reaction is attributed to:

1. Stimulatory effects of tricyclic antidepressants.
2. Changes of neurotransmitter availability and receptor
   sensitivity in the CNS.

Clinical Significance

The value of tricyclic antidepressants for chronic withdrawn schizophrenic patients appears to be small or nil; for
schizophrenic patients with significant depressive symptoms,
the value of tricyclics has not been substantiated. Tricyclic
antidepressants may be contraindicated in some
schizophrenics.

Recommendations

Discontinuation of tricyclic antidepressants is advised if
the schizophrenic condition worsens.

Suggested Readings

Editorial 1980: Use of antidepressants in schizophrenia. *Br Med J* 2:1037–
    1038, 1980.
Kramer, J. C., Klein D. F., Fink M.: Imipramine as an adjunct to
    phenothiazine therapy. *Comp Psychiatry* 3:377–379, 1962.
Pollack M., Klein D. F., Wilkner A., *et al:* Imipramine induced behavioral
    disorganization in schizophrenic patients: Physiologic and psychologic
    correlates. *Recent Adv Biol Psychiatry* 7:53–61, 1965.
Simpson G. M., Amin M., Angus J. W. S., *et al:* Role of antidepressants
    and neuroleptics in the treatment of depression. *Arch Gen Psychiatry*
    27:337–345, 1972.

MISCELLANEOUS EFFECTS

Acne: There is one case report of acne associated with maprotiline. The mechanism suggested is that of an allergic phenomenon.

Ponte C.: Maprotiline-induced acne. *Am J Psychiatry* 139:141, 1982.

Acute renal failure: There are no prior reports of renal failure with tricyclic antidepressants. In a recent report, a 75-year-old woman developed cholestatic jaundice and acute renal failure from treatment with trimipramine, probably the result of an allergic reaction causing acute interstitial nephritis.

Leighton J., Walker R., Lynn K.: Trimipramine-induced acute renal failure. *N Z Med J* 136:248, 1986.

Akathisia: A case of a 20-year-old male who developed akathisia by the third day of treatment with amoxapine for depression is reported. Cogwheel rigidity also developed, along with agitation and restlessness, and these symptoms responded to benztropine.

Ross D. R., Walker J. I., Peterson J.: Akathisia induced by amoxapine. *Am J Psychiatry* 140:115–116, 1983.

Akinesia: A 46-year-old woman was treated for a major depression. Amoxapine was increased from 250 mg/day to 300 mg/day. The patient showed signs of retardation of speech, thought, and movement. Neurological evaluation revealed mild cogwheeling, which responded to medication discontinuation.

Gammon G. D., Hansen C.: A case of akinesia induced by amoxapine. *Am J Psychiatry* 141:283–294, 1984.

Atrial flutter: An 85-year-old male with preexisting cardiac problems was hospitalized for suicidal gestures. He was started on nortriptyline, 25 mg/day, which was increased to 50 mg/day. After 2 weeks, the medication was discontinued because of headaches. After receiving two doses of amoxapine (75 mg/day), he experienced irregular heartbeats and had an ECG that indicated atrial flutter. The drug was discontinued and propranolol started. The ECG returned to normal after 2 days.

Zavodnick S. G.: Atrial flutter with amoxapine: A case report. *Am J Psychiatry* 138(11):1503–1504, 1981.

An 80-year-old female developed atrial flutter after 10 days of maprotiline treatment. The starting dose was 50 mg at bedtime, which was increased to 150 mg/day. The serum concentration was 216 ng/nl before transfer to the CCU.

Tollefon G., Lasae T., Herzog C.: Atrial flutter and maprotiline: Case Report. *J Clin Psychiatry* 45:31–33, 1984.

A 71-year-old female with no previous cardiac fibrillation problems developed atrial fibrillation on a dose of 150 mg/day of amoxapine; the fibrillation subsided after medication discontinuation. In a second case, a 56-year-old male developed atrial fibrillation when the medication was increased from 100 to 150 mg daily of amoxapine.

Murray G. B.: Atrial fibrillation flutter associated with amoxapine: Two case reports. *J Clin Psychopharmacol* 5(2):124–125, 1985.

Cardiac arrhythmia after withdrawal: The patient was withdrawn from 150 mg/day of imipramine. After 19 days, she developed premature ventricular contractions, which subsided after reinstitution of 75 mg/day of imipramine.

Boisvert D., Chouinard G.: Rebound cardiac arrhythmia after withdrawal from imipramine: A case report. *Am J Psychiatry* 138(7):985–986, 1981.

Ejaculatory disturbance: A 33-year-old unmarried male was on a regimen of amoxapine, 50 mg TID, for depression. After 1 day of treatment, the patient complained of no emission of semen and slow and painful muscular contraction. A dosage reduction of amoxapine to 75 mg/day did not decrease sexual dysfunction.

Schwartz G.: Case report of inhibition of ejaculation and retrograde ejaculation as a side effect of amoxapine. *Am J Psychiatry* 139(2):233–234, 1982.

A 29-year-old man with a 2-year history of disabling anxiety and depression was started on amoxapine, 75 mg HS. Painful ejaculation occurred after 3 days and continued to be a problem for 5 weeks, until the drug was discontinued.

Kulik F. A., Wilber R.: Case report of painful ejaculation as a side effect of amoxapine. *Am J Psychiatry* 139(2):234–235, 1982.

Ejaculatory inhibition: There is a case report of trazodone, 100 mg/day, causing ejaculatory inhibition after 1 week of treatment.

Jones S. D.: Ejaculatory inhibition with trazodone. *J Clin Psychopharmacol* 4(5):279–281, 1984.

Emission of semen: There is one case of seminal emission following defecation that is associated with the use of tricyclics.

Breier A., Ginsberg E., Charney D.: Seminal emission induced by tricyclic antidepressants. *Am J Psychiatry* 141:610–611, 1984.

Erythema multiforme: A 63-year-old woman was on trazodone, 300 mg/day, which was increased to 400 mg/day. After 4 days of treatment, she developed a disseminated macular papular eruption with erythematous scale plaques over both hands and the soles of her feet. After 4 days of medication discontinuation, the patient showed a gradual improvement. However, the patient also stopped taking lithium, which has been implicated in dermatological problems.

Ford H. E., Jenike M. A.: Erythema multiforme associated with trazodone therapy: Case report. *J Clin Psychiatry* 46:294–295, 1985.

Galactorrhea: There is one case report of a patient who developed galactorrhea with maprotilene, a side effect that is usually associated with neuroleptics.

Perez O., Henriquez N.: Galactorrhea associated with maprotiline. *Am J Psychiatry* 140:641, 1983.

Hematuria: There are only a few cases that suggest that tricyclics may cause hematuria.

Gillman M., Sandyk R.: Hematuria following tricyclic therapy. *Am J Psychiatry* 141:463–464, 1984.

Hyperglycemia: There is a case report of hyperglycemia in a 49-year-old female on loxapine and lithium for treatment of a bipolar affective disorder. The hyperglycemia developed 5 days after initiation of treatment. On medication discontinuation, the symptoms abated, only to return when amoxapine was reinstated by another psychiatrist.

Tollefson G., Lasar T.: Nonketotic hyperglycemia associated with loxapine and amoxapine: Case report. *J Clin Psychiatry* 44:347–348, 1983.

Increased libido: Three depressed females reported a marked increase of sexual drive during treatment with trazodone and because of this effect were reluctant to discontinue the medication when advised to do so by the psychiatrist.

Gartrell N.: Increased libido in women receiving trazodone. *Am J Psychiatry* 143:781–782, 1986.

Painful postcoital testicular retraction: A letter to the editor reports the occurrence of painful testicular retraction after coitus in a 44-year-old male treated with desipramine. The patient's past history of inguinal hernia may have increased the risk for this adverse effect.

Sorvino A.: Painful postcoital testicular retraction linked with desipramine. *Am J Psychiatry* 143:682–683, 1986.

Perceptual changes: Bupropion was associated with vivid dreaming and changes in attention, memory, and perception in 12 depressed patients. This phenomenon may have resulted from the stimulating and alerting properties of the drug.

Becker R., Dufresne R.: Perceptual changes with bupropion, a novel antidepressant. *Am J Psychiatry* 139:1200–1201, 1982.

Rhabdomyolysis: There is a case report of rhabdomyolysis developing in a 39-year-old woman who ingested approximately 5000 mg amoxapine. The authors speculate that rhabdomyolysis may be caused by direct muscle toxicity or prolonged convulsions or coma.

Abreo K., Shelp W. D., Kosseff A., *et al:* Amoxapine-associated rhabdomyolysis and acute renal failure: Case report. *J Clin Psychiatry* 43(10):426–427, 1982.

Seizure: A 28-year-old male and a 46-year-old female were taking 250 mg/day and 300 mg/day, respectively, of amoxapine. In both cases,

seizures developed 3–4 weeks after therapy was started.
Giannini A. J., Price W. A.: Amoxapine-induced seizures: Case reports. *J Clin Psychiatry* 45:358–359, 1984.

Speech blockage: There are rare reports of speech blockage in patients taking antidepressants such as imipramine, amitriptyline, desipramine, and maprotiline. Speech blockage usually occurs during the first weeks of treatment and responds to reduction in dosage.
Sandyk R.: Speech blockage induced by maprotiline. *Am J Psychiatry* 143:391–392, 1986.

Tardive dyskinesia: The authors describe a case of tardive dyskinesia and parkinsonism in a 49-year-old female treated with amoxapine, 200–300 mg/day, for 8 months. Abnormal movements probably result from the 7–hydroxy metabolite, which has neuroleptic properties.
Thornton, J. E., Stahl S. M.: Case report of tardive dyskinesia and parkinsonism associated with amoxapine therapy. *Am J Psychiatry* 141:704–705, 1984.

Tinnitus (ringing in the ear): There is a case report of protriptyline, 45 mg/day, causing dry mouth and tinnitus, which subsided with dosage reduction. The patient was subsequently changed to desipramine with no return of tinnitus.
Evans D. L., Golden R. N.: Protriptyline and tinnitus. *J Clin Psychopharmacol* 1(6):404–406, 1981.

Vasospasm: There is one well-documented case of vasospasm associated with imipramine, which was established by rechallenge with the drug. Patients who have a history of vasospasm should be monitored for a worsening of the condition when receiving tricyclics.
Appelbaum P., Kapoor W.: Imipramine-induced vasospasm: A case report. *Am J Psychiatry* 140:913–914, 1983.

Ventricular arrhythmias: The study included 20 patients with no preexisting cardiac abnormalities. In two cases, there was a significant increase in premature ventricular contractions. The etiology of ventricular ecotopic beats is unclear. A common denominator in both cases was the presence of mitral valve prolapse.
Janowsky D., Curtis G., Zissook S., *et al:* Trazodone-aggravated ventricular arrhythmias. *J Clin Psychopharmacol* 3(6):372–376, 1983.

Withdrawal dyskinesia: A 63-year-old woman being treated for depression and anxiety received 4 months of amoxapine treatment (250 mg/day), but because of her lack of improvement, the medication was discontinued. After 2 weeks, she noticed involuntary movement of her tongue and lips, which subsided after 10 weeks.
Lesser I.: Case report of withdrawal dyskinesia associated with amoxapine. *Am J Psychiatry* 140:1358–1359, 1983.

3

Reactions to Antidepressants: Monoamine Oxidase Inhibitors

CARDIOVASCULAR EFFECTS

Hypertensive Crisis

Presentation

Hypertensive crisis usually occurs within several hours after ingestion of a contraindicated food or drug. Symptoms include occipital headaches (which may radiate frontally), sore or stiff neck, nausea, vomiting, palpitations (rapid heartbeat), fever, elevated blood pressure, sweating, photophobia (intolerance to light), and dilated pupils. Tachycardia or bradycardia may be present and can be associated with chest pain. With food reactions, factors to be considered include the amount of food eaten, the rate of gastric emptying, and the dose and potency of the monamine oxidase inhibitor (MAOI).

Incidence

Hypertensive crisis is most often associated with ingestion of tyramine-containing foods and sympathomimetic drugs (see Table 1). It is also reported with central nervous system (CNS) depressants, coadministration of other MAOIs, and antidepressants (e.g., imipramine, desipramine). It is most frequently associated with tranylcypromine (structurally related to amphetamine) and less often with phenelzine and isocarboxazid. This reaction may be fatal.

Mechanism

MAOIs irreversibly inhibit the enzyme monoamine oxidase (MAO) in both the central and peripheral nervous systems, which in turn increase presynaptic concentrations of neurotransmitters. Other substances coadministered with an MAOI may potentiate its effects. MAOIs prevent the inactivation of tyramine by MAO in the gut and liver. The excessive amount of tyramine results in the release of norepinephrine from presynaptic storage granules and causes an excessive pressor response. Sympathomimetics (indirect-acting > direct-acting) result in catecholamine release, which in turn allows a larger amount of norepinephrine to react with the receptor.

Table 1. Foods and Drugs Contraindicated for Patients Taking Monoamine Oxidase Inhibitors[a]

Foods	Beverages
Aged cheese[b]	Wine[b]
Pickled herring[b]	Beer[b]
Broad bean pods[b]	Chocolate
Yeast extracts[b]	Coffee
Unfresh fish[b]	Tea
Sour cream	Cola
Yogurt	
Chicken liver	Nonprescription medications
Banana skins	Weight loss products
Avocados	Nasal decongestants
Soy sauce	Cold remedies
Meats with tenderizers	

[a]For a reprint that critically evaluates the 20-plus different diets for MAOIs, write to: Dr. Kenneth I. Shulman, Department of Psychiatry, Sunnybrook Medical Center, 2075 Bayview Avenue, Toronto, Ontario M4N 3M5, Canada.
[b]There is considerable evidence to restrict these nutrients in the diet. In addition, foods that are aged, fermented, smoked, or not fresh should be restricted.

Clinical Significance

It is recommended that these agents not be used in elderly patients or debilitated patients, especially those with a history of hypertension or cardiovascular or cerebrovascular disease. In patients who have a history of frequent or severe headaches, MAOIs may not be the preferred agents to prescribe, since headaches are often the first symptom of an impending hypertensive crisis. It has been reported that intracranial bleeding can occur in association with the hypertension.

The level of inhibition from the MAOI varies with dose and duration of treatment and can persist 2 weeks (with phenelzine) after discontinuation of the drug. With combination MAOI-tricyclic therapy, hypertensive side effects are more often seen if large doses of either agent are used or if the MAOI is initiated prior to the tricyclic antidepressant. More reactions are often seen with the tranylcypromine-imipramine combination. The amine composition of foodstuffs is also unpredictable and variable. It has been recommended that the MAOI diet be continued 1 month after discontinuation of an MAOI.

Recommendations

1. Discontinue the MAOI.
2. Treat hypertension. *Do not use reserpine.* Monitor for rebound hypotension after administering the agent:
   a. Phentolamine, IV
   b. Chlorpromazine, IM/PO
   c. Phenoxybenzamine
3. Apply external cooling to manage fevers.

Suggested Readings

Bethune H. C., Burrell R. H., Culpan R. H., *et al:* Vascular crisis associated with monoamine oxidase inhibitors. *Am J Psychiatry* 3:25–48, 1964.

Blackwell B.: Adverse effects of antidepressant drugs. Part I. *Drugs*
    21:201–219, 1981.
Folks D. G.: Monoamine oxidase inhibitors—Reappraisal of dietary con-
    siderations. *J Clin Psychopharmacol* 3(4):249–252, 1983.
Walker J. I., Davidson J., Zung, W. W.: Patient compliance with MAO
    inhibitor therapy. *J Clin Psychopharmacol* 45(7):78–80, 1984.

Orthostatic Hypotension

Presentation

The presenting signs are light-headedness and
unsteadiness.

The following drug interactions can cause hypotension:

1. Meperidine: This drug will produce rapid onset of
   hypotension and hyperpyrexia—often life-threatening.
   If a narcotic agent is required, morphine, or another
   agent, at low dose can be used with caution.
2. Antihypertensives: Since MAOIs cause hypotension,
   dosage adjustment of the antihypertensives can prevent a severe hypotensive episode.
3. Inhalation anesthesia: Discontinue the MAOI 2 weeks
   prior to elective surgery.

Incidence

The incidence is not known.

Mechanism

The mechanism is not known at this time. The hypotension may result from drug interaction (see Presentation) or a
false transmitter (octopamine).

Clinical Significance

Orthostatic hypotension not due to a drug interaction
will usually subside after a few weeks.

In patients who exhibit hypotension, dosage increases
should be made more gradually.

Recommendations

1. A decrease in the dosage of the MAOI may decrease the severity of hypotension.
2. Hypotension is relieved by having the patient lie down until the blood pressure returns to normal.

Suggested Reading

Walker J. I., Davidson J., Zung W. W.: Patient compliances with MAO inhibitor therapy. *J Clin Psychopharmacol* 45(7):78–80, 1984.

ENDOCRINE EFFECTS

Sexual Dysfunction

Presentation

Inhibited male and female orgasm occurs with phenelzine doses of 15–90 mg/day, most often with a dose of 75 mg/day or more. Dosage decrease has been tried with moderate success. These effects typically occur between the 7th and 8th weeks of drug therapy.

Incidence

Case reports implicate phenelzine in causing inhibition of male and female orgasm. This effect is further supported by a major study in which 111 patients were on phenelzine and 31 patients (22%) experienced this side effect. In contrast, the incidence of inhibited male and female orgasm with tranylcypromine sample is less, but because of the smaller sample size this finding should be interpreted with caution. Other sexual dysfunctions such as decreased libido and erectile dysfunction have been noted in case reports, but appear to be very infrequent.

Mechanism

The physiology for this group of reactions is similar to the proposed mechanism for tricyclic and tetracyclic antidepressants; i.e., MAOIs affect the autonomic nervous system and the hypothalamic–pituitary–gonadal axis.

Clinical Significance

The impairment of sexual dysfunction may be a symptom of depression. However, depression usually leads to disorders of sexual desire, rather than alteration in function. Before considering drug discontinuation in an otherwise responsive patient, it may be wise to continue the medication to see whether this symptom persists. If the patient continues to have this problem after additional time, a change should be considered to prevent compliance problems.

Recommendations

1. Obtain a complete sexual history.
2. Rule out organic problems that could cause sexual dysfunction.
3. Decrease the dosage if possible.
4. Change to a nonhydraxine MAOI.
5. Bethanechol, up to 50 mg daily, can be added.

Suggested Readings

Christenson R.: MAOIs, anorgasmia, and weight gain (letter). *Am J Psychiatry* 140(9):1260, 1983.

Lesko L. M., Stotland W. L., Segraves R. T.: Three cases of female anorgasmia associated with MAOIs. *Am J Psychiatry* 139(10):1353–1354, 1982.

Mitchell J. E., Popkin M. K.: Antidepressant drug therapy and sexual dysfunction in men. A review. *J Clin Psychopharmacol* 3(2):76–79, 1983.

Rabkin J. G., Quitkin F. M., McGrath P., *et al:* Adverse reactions to monoamine oxidase inhibitors. Part II. Treatment correlates and clinical management. *J Clin Psychopharmacol* 5(1):2–9, 1985.

Shen W. W., Mallya A. R.: MAOI-induced inhibited female orgasm (letter). *Am J Psychiatry* 140(9):1275, 1983.

Weight Gain

Presentation

Weight gain with phenelzine can occur over a 3-month period; the longer the duration of treatment, the greater the weight gain. One patient was noted to have a 25-pound weight gain over 26 weeks. Lowering the dose of phenelzine is not associated with weight loss.

Incidence

The incidence of weight gain appears to be primarily associated with phenelzine, reported in a retrospective study to occur in 10% of the patients. Case reports also mention weight gain with phenelzine. The incidence with tranylcypromine and isocarboxazid is negligible. In fact, one paper suggests that isocarboxazid should be used in patients who gain weight from other MAOIs.

Mechanism

The specific mechanism is unclear and requires more research. The few postulated mechanisms involve either metabolic alteration, specific neurotransmitters that may regulate eating behavior, or both.

Clinical Significance

Depressive disorders may contribute to overeating and a concern about weight gain in about 14% of the patients. Phenelzine appears to cause weight increase, which may affect medication compliance.

Recommendations

1. Avoid phenelzine in obese patients.
2. If a change in MAOI is needed, use isocarboxazid.

One study using isocarboxazid caused a weight reduction over a 2- to 4-week period.
3. Monitor weight at scheduled appointments.

Suggested Readings

Christenson, R.: MAOI's, anorgasmia, and weight gain. *Am J Psychiatry* 140(9):1260, 1983.

Davidson J., Turnbull, C.: Loss of appetite and weight associated with monoamine oxidase inhibitor isocarboxazid. *J Clin Psychopharmacol* 2(4):263–266, 1982.

Paykel E. S.: Depression and appetite. *J Psychosom Res* 21:401–407, 1977.

Rabkin J. G., Quitkin F. M., McGrath P., *et al:* Adverse reactions to monoamine oxidase inhibitors. *J Clin Psychopharmacol* 5(1):2–9, 1985.

HEPATIC EFFECTS

Presentation

Hepatotoxic jaundice may develop within a few months of starting an MAOI, or it may not appear until after several years of treatment. Jaundice may be accompanied by pyrexia (fever) and vomiting, and the liver may be tender and palpable. Liver function tests, including serum transaminases, bilirubin, and alkaline phosphatase, would be elevated. Morgan and Reed (1972) found that patients with cirrhosis are likely to exhibit marked sensitivity to tranylcypromine (slow electroencephalographic activity and obtunded consciousness), and there is particular risk if there is also a history of previous hepatic encephalopathy.

Incidence

Hepatotoxic reactions were more common with the older hydrazine derivatives (iproniazid and pheniprazine), which have been withdrawn from the market. There are only a few case reports involving phenelzine, so the reaction appears to be rare. Severe liver damage may be less likely with tranylcypromine, but this drug has been used less often and studied less than phenelzine.

Mechanism

Development of jaundice appears to involve diffuse hepatocellular damage; this damage has also been attributed to a hypersensitivity type of reaction. The one case of angiosarcoma associated with phenelzine appears to implicate a carcinogenic mechanism.

Clinical Significance

Both phenelzine and tranylcypromine are unlikely to cause liver damage unless there is a history of previous hepatic toxicity such as might result from hepatitis or alcoholic or other drug-induced liver disease that remains unresolved. In normal, healthy patients, the risk of hepatic reactions is indeed very low. Clinicians should be aware that phenelzine may cause methodological interference with the SMA 12/60 method that may result in overestimation of serum bilirubin and that phenelzine can also cause decreases in serum cholinesterase.

Recommendations

If there is evidence of hepatic toxicity, MAOIs should be discontinued immediately and proper medical treatment instituted. A careful medical history and predrug base-line liver function tests may help to identify patients at risk for hepatotoxic reactions.

Suggested Readings

Cook G. C., Sherlock S.: Jaundice and its relation to therapeutic agents. *Lancet* 1:175–179, 1965.

Daneshmend T. K., Scott G. L., Bradfield J. W.: Antidepressants and liver damage associated with phenelzine. *Br Med J* 1:1679, 1979.

Morgan M., Reed A.: Antidepressants and liver disease. *Gut* 13:697–701, 1972.

Sher P. Drug interference with laboratory test: Bilirubin. *Drug Ther*
    1976:153–156, 1976.

NEUROLOGICAL EFFECTS

Hypomania

Presentation

Behavioral changes consist of agitation, sleeplessness,
irritability, euphoria, hyperactivity, talkativeness, intrusiveness, and other manic symptoms.

The earliest latency to onset of manic/hypomanic symptoms is about 2–3 weeks. Chronic administration of MAOIs
produces an increased severity of manic/hypomanic symptoms and a significant shortened latency to time of onset.

Incidence

The incidence among patients with bipolar disorder is
about 35%; among patients with unipolar disorder, it is very
low, about 4.5%.

Mechanism

Suggested mechanisms for neurological reaction include
increased CNS activity of amine neurotransmitters of their
metabolites and possible changes in postsynaptic receptor
supersensitivity.

Clinical Significance

The "switch process" is more common in patients with
a history of manic/hypomanic episodes than in patients
without such a history.

Recommendations

1. Very low doses of MAOIs used in combination with lithium carbonate are recommended in patients with bipolar illness.
2. Discontinue MAOIs when manic symptoms are present.
3. Lithium salts alone may have a more satisfactory outcome with a more stable course in some cases.

Suggested Readings

Pickar D., Murphy D. L., Cohen R. M., Campbell I. C., Lipper S.: Selective and nonselective monoamine oxidase inhibitors. *Arch Gen Psychiatry* 39:535–540, 1982.

Bunney W. E.: Psychopharmacology of the switch process in affective disorders, in Lipton M. A., DiMascio A., Killman K. F. (eds): *Psychopharmacology: A Generation of Progress.* New York, Raven Press, 1978, pp 1249–1259.

Paresthesias

Presentation

The presenting picture may be one of peripheral neuropathy, including tingling sensations of the feet and hands and the "electric-shock-like" sensations that occur on turning the head or eyes. Carpal tunnel syndrome (a type of numbness in the hands or fingers) has also been reported.

Incidence

Vitamin B_6 deficiency may occur in only a small percentage of patients treated with MAOIs and may be dose-related. Malnourished patients and patients who are predisposed to neuritis (e.g., diabetics and alcoholics) are most susceptible to this drug-induced deficiency state. Long-term usage of MAOIs may also increase the risks of developing paresthesias.

Mechanism

MAOIs can produce pyridoxine (vitamin B_6) deficiency. A hydrazine drug such as phenelzine combines with the aldehyde group of pyridoxal phosphate, which then becomes physiologically inactive. An amine drug such as tranylcypromine combines with the aldehyde of pyridoxal phosphate and forms an imine (Schiff base).

Clinical Significance

Appropriate medical management with pyridoxine supplementation usually prevents such side effects.

Recommendations

Prescribe pyridoxine (vitamin B_6), 300 mg daily.

Suggested Readings

Harrison W., Stewart J., Lovelace R., Quitkin F.: Case report of carpal tunnel syndrome associated with tranylcypromine. *Am J Psychiatry* 140:1229–1230, 1983.

Raskin N. H., Fishman R. A.: Pyridoxine deficiency neuropathy due to hydralazine. *N Engl J Med* 273:1182–1185, 1965.

Sheedham D., Claycomb J. B., Koureta N.: Monoamine oxidase inhibitors: Prescription and patient management. *Int J Psychiatry Med* 10:99–121, 1980–1981.

Stimulant Effects

Presentation

There is a sudden increase in agitation, motor restlessness, anxiety, irritability, and insomnia. Insomnia is a common complaint in patients on MAOIs, especially when the drug is administered late in the day or evening.

Mechanism

The mechanism is one of direct stimulatory effect of MAOIs on the CNS, leading to alteration of neurotramsmitter activity and receptor sensitivity in the CNS.

Clinical Significance

1. This reaction may cause poor medication compliance.
2. Usually, patients fall asleep without difficulty but suffer from mid or terminal insomnia (i.e., they wake up in the middle of the night or close to morning).
3. Usually, CNS stimulant effects are of little clinical significance. They are readily alleviated by any or a combination of dose reduction, a change in dosing regimen, and supportive measures.

Recommendations

1. If the symptoms are severe, discontinue the MAOI.
2. Avoid prescribing nighttime doses.
3. Start the drug at a lower dose and increase the dose gradually.

Suggested Readings

Zisook, S.: Side effect of isocarboxazid. *J Clin Psychiatry* 45:53–58, 1984.
Zisook, S.: A clinical overview of monoamine oxidase inhibitors. *Psychosomatics* 26:240–251, 1985.

WITHDRAWAL EFFECTS

Presentation

In addition to symptoms reported by Tyrer (see Incidence), there are reports of muscle weakness, tremulousness, vivid and frightening nightmares, intense frontal headache, shivering, irritability, paresthesias, and myoclonic jerking.

Liskin *et al* (1985) reported two cases of an acute organic psychosis marked by visual, auditory, and tactile hallucinations after abrupt discontinuation of phenelzine. The onset of withdrawal effects has been reported to occur 24 hr after discontinuation of MAOIs; in the two cases reported by Liskin and co-workers, the symptoms gradually worsened over a 3- to 4-day period.

Incidence

There are only a handful of case reports, which range in the severity of withdrawal symptoms. Tyrer (1984) reported that almost 30% of patients discontinuing phenelzine experienced either palpitations, nausea, sweating, or depersonalization. In a rapid eye movement (REM) sleep study, two of four patients who stopped MAOIs became profoundly anxious.

Mechanism

Withdrawal effects have been related to MAOI supression of REM sleep. After discontinuation of an MAOI, REM sleep rebounds as much as 250% above normal levels. However, it is not known whether this mechanism could account for all the symptoms observed after abrupt MAOI withdrawal.

Clinical Significance

Severe withdrawal reactions are probably highly unlikely, but milder reactions may be experienced by patients who abruptly discontinue MAOIs. The clinician should keep withdrawal effects in mind, since a withdrawal reaction may be misdiagnosed as the reappearance of previously controlled symptoms. There is speculation that if a patient experiences withdrawal-like symptoms (such as myoclonic jerks, paresthesias, and hypnopompic hallucinations) during the course of treatment with an MAOI, he may be at a higher risk for similar symptoms after abrupt withdrawal. MAOIs not infrequently cause unacceptable side effects during treatment, which may lead the patient to abruptly discontinue medication. If the patient has received usual or higher doses for 1 month or more, the clinician should caution the patient concerning the possibility of withdrawal reactions.

Recommendations

Withdrawal reactions are best prevented by tapering MAOIs gradually (over 2 weeks). In some case reports of severe withdrawal reactions, the drug has been reinstituted and then slowly tapered. Most withdrawal reactions, however, will probably be mild and require no treatment other than patient reassurance.

Suggested Readings

Liskin B., Roose S. P., Walsh B. T.: Acute psychosis following phenelzine discontinuation. *J Clin Psychopharmacol* 5:46–47, 1985.

Palladino A.: Adverse reactions to abrupt discontinuation of phenelzine. *J Clin Psychopharmacol* 3:3206–3207, 1983.

Tyrer P.: Clinical effects of abrupt withdrawal from tricyclic antidepressants and monoamine oxidase inhibitors after long-term treatment. *J Affect Dis* 6:1–7, 1984.

Wyatt R., Fram D. H., Kuper D. J., *et al:* Total prolonged drug-induced REM sleep supression in anxious–depressed patients. *Arch Gen Psychiatry* 24:145–155, 1971.

MISCELLANEOUS EFFECTS

Leukopenia: Leukopenia is a very rare, but potentially serious, side effect of MAOIs.

Tipermas A., Gilman, Russakoff M.: A case report of leukopenia associated with phenelzine. *Am J. Psychiatry* 141:806–807, 1984.

Nightmares: Two cases of nightmares occurred 2–3 days after the dosage of phenelzine was altered by the patients. In the first case, a 70-year-old female who abruptly stopped taking 60 mg/day of phenelzine began experiencing nightmares 8 days after medication withdrawal. In the second case, a 28-year-old male was taking 90 mg/day of phenelzine. He decreased his dose to 60 mg/day; after 10 days, he began experiencing nightmares. In both cases, the patient had a relapse of depression in 2 weeks.

Joyce P. R., Walshe J.: Nightmares during phenelzine withdrawal. *J Clin Psychopharmacol* 3(2):121, 1983.

Parkinsonian side effects: An elderly depressed woman developed parkinsonian syndrome with phenelzine. This is apparently the first report of such symptoms with MAOIs.

Teusink J., Alexopoulos G., Shamoian C.: Parkinsonian side effects induced by a MAO inhibitor. *Am J Psychiatry* 141:118–119, 1984.

A subsequent case was reported in a 42-year-old woman; the onset of parkinsonian symptoms was noted 5 weeks after phenelzine was started.

Gillman M. A., Sandyk R.: Parkinsonism induced by a monoamine oxidase inhibitor. *Postgrad Med J* 62:235–236, 1986.

4

Reactions to Lithium

DERMATOLOGICAL EFFECTS

Presentation

Maculopapular eruptions are usually generalized and pruritic (itchy). The eruptions will clear with or without discontinuing or reducing the dosage of lithium or administering antihistamines or topical steroids.

Acneiform eruptions: Lithium can cause or exacerbate acneiform eruptions. There is no treatment that is consistently effective. It may be necessary to decrease the dose or discontinue therapy completely.

Alopecia (hair loss): There are more frequent reports of hair loss with lithium beginning to appear in the literature. The condition is reversible following discontinuation of lithium.

Follicular eruptions: These are often hyperkeratotic, erythematous follicular papules. They are of limited distribution and asymptomatic. They may remit spontaneously with continued lithium therapy. There are a limited number of reports in the literature, but such eruptions may be a common occurrence in lithium-treated patients.

Psoriasis: Exacerbation of existing psoriasis is common, is quite resistant to usual treatments, and may require discontinuation of the lithium for the condition to clear.

Other reactions reported (isolated reports) are exfoliative dermatitis, generalized pruritis and erythema (redness); alopecia (hair loss), dermatitis herpetiformis, stomatitis (inflammation of the mouth), ichthyosis (dry, scaly skin), xerosis (abnormal dryness of the skin and mucous membranes in conjunctiva).

Incidence

Onset is variable, occurring within days or weeks after the initiation of lithium and even months to years later after continued therapy. One study comparing a lithium-treated group and a non-lithium-treated group reported a 34% overall incidence of cutaneous reactions possibly induced by lithium (Dimocritos *et al*, 1983). This same study suggested that females may be more predisposed to develop dermatological reactions than males.

Mechanism

The exact mechanism of lithium-induced skin reactions is not well understood, but may be related to serum levels. However, none of the reactions is due to toxic levels, but a decrease in serum levels can lead to improvement if dermatological reactions are present.

For lithium-induced psoriasis, there are two suggested mechanisms: (1) lithium's ability to inhibit the adenyl-cyclase–cyclic AMP (cAMP) system, thereby reducing the accumulation of cAMP in epidermal cells—it has been demonstrated that there is a reduced amount of cAMP in psoriatic skin; (2) an indirect mechanism whereby lithium induces proliferation and sensitization of polymorphonuclear leukocytes.

Clinical Significance

It is possible that patients with (or predisposed to) skin disorders are likely to develop exacerbations of eruptions. Practically all the lithium-induced skin reactions are reversible after discontinuation of the drug.

Recommendations

1. If specific topical therapy does not alleviate the eruption, a dosage reduction should be tried if possible.
2. Discontinuation of lithium should be the last choice if serious eruptions continue. The risk vs. benefit of discontinuing medication should be carefully reviewed.

Maculopapular rash: Continue the therapy and see whether eruptions clear spontaneously. Topical steroids and antihistamines can be used for symptomatic treatment.

Acneiform eruptions: Try topical acne preparations, i.e., drying agents, topical antibiotics.

Psoriasis: Try the standard treatments (e.g., topical steroids); discontinue lithium or switch to carbamazepine if psoriasis is severe or unresponsive to treatments.

Suggested Readings

Deandrea D., Walker N., Mehlmauer M., *et al:* Dermatological reactions to lithium: A critical review of the literature. *J Clin Psychopharmacol* 2(3):199–203, 1982.

Dimocritos S., Waters B.: A review of controlled study of cutaneous conditions associated with lithium carbonate. *Br J Psychiatry* 143:42–50, 1983.

Orwin A.: Hair loss following lithium therapy. *Br. J. Dermatol.* 108:503, 1983.

Skott A.: Lithium and psoriasis (letter). *Br J Psychiatry* 131:223, 1977.

CARDIOVASCULAR EFFECTS

Presentation

There are three known categories of cardiac effects: electrocardiographic (ECG) changes that are benign (T-wave flattening or inversion), disturbances in impulse formation and conduction (sick sinus syndrome, sinus node abnormalities and sinoatrial or atrioventricular block, ventricular tachycardia and fibrillation, multiple premature ventricular contractions), and structural or myocardial abnormalities (myocarditis, myocardial infarction, and cardiac malformations in infants whose mothers received lithium during pregnancy). Lithium toxicity produces ECG changes similar to those noted above, but ST segment depression and Q–T interval prolongation have also been noted. There are also case reports of conduction defects and myocardial abnormalities that have occurred during lithium intoxication.

Incidence

Benign ECG changes in the T wave are commonly observed in 20–30% of patients receiving lithium. Conduction disturbances, such as arrhythmias, have been reported less frequently. There are only a few case reports involving myocardial abnormalities. Cardiac malformation in the fetus (Ebstein's anomaly) during pregnancy occurred in 11 of 143 babies, but the true incidence may be lower because of overreporting in lithium registries.

Mechanism

Benign ECG changes resemble the effects of hypokalemia, so it is thought that lithium may be replacing potassium in the myocardium. Another mechanism may be lithium's ability to interfere with epinephrine's stimulation of adenylcyclase, thus blunting the action of epinephrine in the myocardium.

Clinical Significance

The significance of ECG changes is not known, but most experts consider them to be benign, and their appearance would not be considered a contraindication to continuing treatment. These ECG effects are also seen with neuroleptics and tricyclic antidepressants and are considered to be benign and asymptomatic, usually appearing early after lithium is started. Disturbances in impulse formation and conduction defects are much less commonly seen, but need careful evaluation if they appear. Some of these problems, particularly cardiac arrhythmias, represent lithium's exacerbation of a preexisting condition. These changes may be more likely to occur in older persons with preexisting cardiac disease. Myocardial abnormalities appear to be very rare. All three categories of cardiac effects can occur with lithium intoxication and may be more pronounced. Since lithium has been implicated in the development of specific cardiac malformation during pregnancy, it should be avoided during the first trimester if possible.

Recommendations

Although lithium generally produces benign and reversible cardiac effects, one should carefully review cardiac status before prescribing lithium. In patients over the age of 40 years, a baseline ECG should be obtained and repeated once a year during treatment. If there are any preexisting cardiac conditions, consultation with a specialist should be sought. Although infrequent, disturbances in impulse formation and cardiac conduction may lead to complaints of palpitations and alteration in consciousness. These symptoms should receive careful evaluation. If lithium intoxication occurs, the patient's cardiac status should be monitored.

Suggested Readings

Jefferson J. W., Greist J. H., Ackerman D. L.: Cardiovascular effects, in: *Lithium Encyclopedia for Clinical Practice*. Washington, DC, American Psychiatric Press, 1983, pp 85–86.
Mitchell J. E., Mackenzie T. B.: Cardiac effects of lithium therapy in man: A review. *J Clin Psychiatry* 43:47–51, 1982.

GASTROINTESTINAL EFFECTS

Presentation

Signs of gastrointestinal (GI) upset include nausea, vomiting, anorexia, loose stools, and abdominal pains. There are only a few reports of gastric ulcers that occurred during lithium therapy.

Incidence

GI effects are common in the initial stages of lithium therapy; in one report, 30% of patients experienced such symptoms in the first 2 weeks of therapy, but no GI upset was found 1 year later (Schou *et al*, 1970).

Mechanism

There are two mechanisms thought to be responsible for the gastrointestinal effects of lithium: unabsorbed lithium in the intestine may give rise to diarrhea or loose stools; and rapid absorption of lithium (particularly high plasma peaks) is usually associated with complaints of nausea and vomiting.

Clinical Significance

Abdominal symptoms appear to be common and must be expected in approximately one third of patients early in treatment. They are usually mild in nature and occur with serum levels that are within the normal range. However, it is important that the clinician pay close attention to such symptoms, since they are also associated with lithium intoxication.

One should be very cautious about prescribing lithium for a patient with a GI condition.

Recommendations

In most cases, reassure the patient that GI effects are temporary in nature. They can be minimized, however, by changing either the dosage schedule or the preparation in cases that are more severe but not related to toxicity. Symptoms related to the peak level can be minimized by giving lithium in divided doses during the day and by directing that the lithium be taken with meals to slow absorption, or the long-acting oral dosage form such as Lithobid®. In cases of severe GI distress, it may be necessary to lower the dosage or temporarily discontinue lithium if possible.

Suggested Readings

Cooper T. B., Simpson G. M., Lee J. H., *et al:* Evaluation of a slow-release lithium carbonate formulation. *Am J Psychiatry* 135:917–922, 1978.

Mattsson A., Seltzer R. L.: Lithium carbonate and gastric ulcer. *Am J Psychiatry* 138:124, 1981.

Schou M., Baastrup P. C., Grof P., *et al:* Pharmacological and clinical problems of lithium prophylaxis. *Br J Psychiatry* 116:615–619, 1970.

HEMATOLOGICAL EFFECTS (LEUKOCYTOSIS)

Presentation

Leukocyte counts are most elevated during the first few weeks of lithium therapy. Increases in the mean value of leukocytes are around $10,000/mm^3$, ranging, rarely, up to $25,000/mm^3$.

Leukocytosis is not related to age, sex, or psychiatric diagnosis; serum lithium levels above 0.5 meq/liter are required for this effect, but there is no proportional response to dose. This effect is reversible, usually returning to base-line level within 7–10 days after lithium is discontinued.

Incidence

Mild to moderate leukocytosis is not an uncommon phenomenon in patients receiving lithium therapy. Elevation to about $10,000/mm^3$ persisted in 66% of patients at the 1-year and 68% at the 2-year follow-up (Pi *et al,* 1983).

Mechanism

Leukocytosis is mediated by increased production of colony-stimulating factor and subsequent proliferation of my-eloid cells. Leukocytosis is characterized by an increase in neutrophils and is thought to derive from increased gran-ulocyte production rather than from a redistribution of granulocytes.

Clinical Significance

Lithium-induced leukocytosis is usually benign. Once other possible causes of leukocytosis (such as infection) are ruled out, there is little clinical significance to a moderately elevated white count. It has been reported that lithium may be useful as a therapeutic agent for increasing the granulocyte counts in patients with leukopenia and aplastic anemia (Pi and Dempsey, 1983).

Recommendations

Clinicians should keep the common finding of lithium-induced leukocytosis in mind when conducting routine medical work-ups on lithium-treated patients.

Suggested Readings

Hammond W. P., Dale D. C.: Cyclic hematopoiesis: Effects of lithium on colony-forming cells and colony-stimulating activity in grey collie dogs. *Blood* 59:179–184, 1982.

Jefferson J. W., Greist J. H., Ackerman D. L.: *Lithium Encyclopedia for Clinical Practice.* Washington, DC, American Psychiatric Press, 1983.

Murphy D. L., Goodwin F. K., Bunney W. E.: Leukocytosis during lithium treatment. *Am J Psychiatry* 127:1559–1561, 1971.

Pi E. H., Dempsey G. M.: Lithium carbonate in aplastic anemia. *Arch Gen Psychiatry* 37:720, 1980.

Pi E. H., Sramek J. J., Simpson G. M.: Effect of lithium on leukocytes: A two-year follow-up. *J Clin Psychiatry* 44:139–140, 1983.

Stein R. S., Hanson G., Koether S., *et al.:* Lithium-induced granulocytosis. *Ann Intern Med* 88:809–810, 1978.

RENAL EFFECTS

Diabetes Insipidus and Polyuria

Presentation

Symptoms of polyuria (frequent urination) usually occur after lithium therapy is initiated. This reaction usually diminishes after a few days; however, in some cases, it may persist for as long as a few weeks. In addition, the patient will also develop polydipsia (increased fluid intake) to compensate for the fluid loss. Occasionally, the polydipsia and polyuria may progress to diabetes insipidus with constant thirst, frequent urination, and an inability to concentrate urine in response to water deprivation.

Incidence

Polyuria is a common side effect of lithium therapy and occurs in 40% of patients. In approximately 12% of patients, polyuria may continue progressing to diabetes insipidus.

Mechanism

Polyuria and diabetes insipidus are associated with an inhibitory effect on the antidiuretic hormone (ADH) in the renal tubules. This effect is not a central nervous system (CNS) deficiency of ADH, but occurs mainly in the kidneys. Supplementation with ADH is not particularly effective, however.

Clinical Significance

Polyuria is usually well tolerated and does not lead to other medical problems. Diabetes insipidus can exacerbate polydipsia, leading to frequent intake of fluids with accompanying weight gain. This may exacerbate medical problems such as congestive heart failure and hypertension. In addition, frequent urination leads to altered sleep pattern.

Recommendations

1. Question the patient about polyuria, polydipsia, and nocturia (urination at night) and when these symptoms occurred.
2. Perform a water deprivation test.
3. Check urine osmolality and specific gravity.

4. If diabetes insipidus is confirmed, one can give 25–
50 mg hydrochlorthiazine (HCT). However, the long-
term effects of HCT are unknown. (Note: If HCT
therapy is initiated, the lithium dose should be decreased by 50% and lithium levels should be
monitored carefully to reestablish the maintenance
lithium dosage.) A recent report indicates that the
new diuretic amiloride is helpful in treating lithium-
induced diabetes insipidus.

Suggested Readings

Baldessarini R. J., Lipinski J. F., Lithium salts 1970–1975. *Ann Intern
Med* 83:527–533, 1975.
Jefferson, J. W., Greist J. H.: *Primer of Lithium Therapy*. Baltimore,
Williams & Wilkins, 1977, pp 151–159.
Koster T. R., Forrest J. N.: Treatment of severe lithium-induced polyuria
with amiloride. *Am. J. Psychiatry* 143:1563–1568, 1986.
Ramsey T. A., Cox M.: Lithium and the kidney: A review. *Am J
Psychiatry* 139(4):443–449, 1982.
Singer I., Forrest J. N.: Drug-induced states of nephrogenic diabetes
insipidus. *Kidney Int* 10:82–95, 1976.

Structural Damage (Nephrotoxicity)

Presentation

The patient may complain of frequent urination. There is
some evidence that patients with frequent urination (polyuria)
may have a predisposition to this reaction. However, on the
basis of the available data, this conclusion must be interpreted as tentative.

Incidence

No specific information on the incidence of this reaction
is available. Many clinicians consider this a very infrequent
complication of lithium therapy. From a review of the
literature on lithium-induced kidney damage, it appears that
patients with histories of lithium intoxication may have a
higher incidence. In addition, the reports are complicated by

methodological problems, raising doubts about whether such lesions are due exclusively to lithium.

Mechanism

Lithium therapy has been associated with tubular atrophy, interstitial fibrosis, and sclerotic glomeruli in the kidney. The mechanism in man is at present unknown. Animal studies show damage in the mitochondria of the distal portion of the nephron. Whether lithium salts are nephrotoxic in humans is still controversial.

Clinical Significance

The initiation of lithium maintenance therapy should include a consideration of lithium's possible nephrotoxic effects. However, the mortality and morbidity from manic–depressive illness are significant. Considering the studies available, only a small percentage of patients develop structural damage. Patients who derive significant benefits from lithium therapy should not be precluded from its use.

Recommendations

1. Complete medical history.
2. Drug history (possible exposure to nephrotoxins).
3. Lowest effective lithium dose (response with levels as low as 0.4 meq/liter is sometimes possible).
4. Periodic lab tests (serum creatinine, electrolytes, fluid deprivation, urine specific gravity) to monitor renal status.

Suggested Readings

Hwang S., Tuason V. B.: Long-term maintenance lithium therapy and possible irreversible renal damage. *J Clin Psychiatry* 41(1):11–19, 1980.

Jenner F. A.: Lithium and the question of kidney damage. *Arch Gen Psychiatry* 36:888–890, 1979.

Lippman S.: Is lithium bad for the kidneys? *J Clin Psychiatry* 43(6):220–224, 1982.

Ramsey T. A., Cox M.: Lithium and the kidney: A review. *Am J Psychiatry* 139(4):443–449, 1982.

TERATOGENIC EFFECTS

Presentation

The vast majority of malformations reported by Weinstein and Goldfield (1975) were abnormalities of the heart and great vessels, including an overrepresentative number of the rare Ebstein's anomaly. Other malformations included single umbilical artery, anomalies of the CNS, malformed external ears, Down's syndrome, intracerebral toxoplasmosis, and stillbirth.

Incidence

In babies whose mothers had taken lithium during the first 3 months of pregnancy, the incidences of congenital malformation ranged from 9.1% (13/143) to 11.1% (25/225).

Mechanism

The mechanism is unknown.

Clinical Significance

Although teratogenicity of lithium in humans is undetermined, reports suggest that lithium may be a teratogen in the cardiovascular system.

Recommendations

Lithium should not be given to pregnant women during the first trimester. For some cases, when physicians consider that the risk of relapse of affective episode may outweigh the risk of possible teratogenicity of lithium during early pregnancy, such treatment decisions must be individualized, justified, and carefully documented. If it is necessary to continue lithium treatment, the lowest possible serum level should be maintained.

Suggested Readings

Jefferson J. W., Greist J. H., Ackerman D. L.: *Lithium Encyclopedia for Clinical Practice*. Washington, DC, American Psychiatric Press, 1983, pp 264–265.

Weinstein M. R., Goldfield M. D.: Cardiovascular malformations with lithium use during pregnancy. *Am J Psychiatry* 132:529, 1975.

THYROID EFFECTS (HYPOTHYROIDISM)

Presentation

During long-term treatment, euthyroid patients can develop a goiter or hypothyroidism with or without goiter. A change in thyroid function tests will often occur before the presentation of clinical symptoms. Thyroid function test alterations are seen early in treatment:

1. Thyroxine (T_4) and triiodothyronine (T_3) levels are lowered.
2. Thyroid-stimulating hormone (TSH) level is elevated.
3. TSH-releasing hormone (TRH) stimulation of TSH is the most sensitive parameter.

Incidence

Thyroid effects are more common in females greater than 40 years of age.

Of patients on long-term lithium therapy, 5–15% have either altered thyroid function tests or clinical symptoms.

Mechanism

Human and animal studies show that lithium has an inhibitory effect on the thyroid gland, resulting in a decrease in hormone secretion. Another possible mechanism (especially for development of goiter) is lithium-induced autoimmune thyroiditis. The significance of antithyroid antibodies is questionable, since one can have high levels of antibodies without hypothyroidism and hypothyroidism can occur without antithyroid antibodies.

Clinical Significance

Hypothyroidism may occur more frequently in patients predisposed to thyroid disorders. There has been no relationship demonstrated with serum levels, duration of treatment, or the concurrent use of other psychotropic drugs. One study shows the usual decrease in T_4 and T_3 and increase in TSH early in therapy, but from months 4 to 12, unexpectedly, T_4 and T_3 increased to pretreatment levels, and TSH decreased but was still above pretreatment levels (Sinagan *et al*, 1984). This suggests a possible spontaneous improvement of thyroid function with continued therapy. In most cases, the changes in thyroid function tests are not significant enough to require treatment. If necessary, thyroid supplementation may be administered. Hyperthyroidism has been reported in lithium-treated patients, but is rarely seen.

Recommendations

1. Take base-line thyroid function tests before initiating lithium treatment. Repeat the tests in 4 months. If an abnormal value is obtained, repeat the test.
2. If thyroid hormone supplement is necessary, levothyroxine is often the agent of choice.
3. Underlying thyroid disorders are not an absolute contraindication to lithium treatment if thyroid function can be properly monitored.

Suggested Readings

Amdisen A., Anderson C. J.: Lithium treatment and thyroid function. *Pharmacopsychiatry* 15:149–155, 1982.

Sinagan L., Wahlin A., Jacobsson L., *et al:* Lithium therapy and thyroid function tests. *Neuropsychobiology* 11(1):39–43, 1984.

Vestergaard P.: Clinically important side effects of long-term lithium treatment: A review. *Acta Psychiatr Scand (Suppl)* 305:1–36, 1983.

TREMOR

Presentation

Lithium-induced tremor is an action-based tremor. The patient complains of exacerbation of the tremor in performing specific tasks. For example, a female may have difficulty applying her make-up or a barber may have difficulty in cutting hair. This tremor is not a resting tremor as seen with neuroleptic use.

Lithium-induced postural tremor is much more pronounced than the tremor seen at rest. Lithium tremor has irregular rhythm and amplitude and is jerky. It is more apparent in the fingers. The movement is not rotational, but more of flexion and extension of the fingers with occasionally side movements. The frequency of the tremor is 6–12 Hz.

Incidence

Tremor is commonly seen after initiating lithium therapy and after chronic therapy. The incidence in chronic therapy is reported to be as high as 65%. It may occur more often in men and the elderly.

Mechanism

Lithium tremor is thought to be of peripheral, not central, origin. Lithium may be overstimulating β-receptors in skeletal muscle, perhaps directly or by catecholamine imbalance.

Clinical Significance

There does not appear to be an association between the occurrence of tremor and the duration of treatment. The tremor is related to dosage or serum levels and is less severe than the coarse tremor seen with lithium toxicity. Tremor induced by lithium is more frequently seen in patients with a familial history of essential tremor. An increased frequency of tremor has been noted in patients on both lithium and a tricyclic antidepressant.

Lithium tremor can be differentiated from parkinsonian tremor in that parkinsonian has slower, rhythmic, rotational flexing movements. Parkinsonian tremor involves fingers, hand, and wrist as a unit, with less postural tremor; on action, the slow resting tremor becomes faster in frequency.

Resting tremor is a characteristic feature, and the action
tremor is significant. Lithium tremor is differentiated from
essential tremor in that essential tremor is characteristically a
contraction tremor, and is not jerky, but smoother and
rhythmic. A therapeutic effect of propranolol treatment on
lithium tremor can be seen in 30–60 min.

Recommendations

1. On the basis of the proposed mechanism, a β-
   blocker, such as propranolol, can be used. Doses
   range from 30 to 80 mg/day (it is usually not
   necessary to exceed 40 mg/day). In case reports,
   tremor was completely controlled with propranolol
   and recurred when propranolol was discontinued.
2. In patients who could not use propranolol due to
   history of bronchospasm, metoprolol (a selective β-
   blocker) has been used successfully at doses of 25–
   50 mg BID.
3. Other β-blockers have been utilized—nadolol, oxy-
   prenolol, pindolol.

Suggested Readings

Gaby N. S., Lefkowitz D. S., Israel J. R.: Treatment of lithium tremor
    with metoprolol. *Am J Psychiatry* 140(5):593–595, 1983.
Lapierre Y. D.: Control of lithium tremor with propranolol. *Can Med
    Assoc J* 114:619–620, 1976.
Pullinger S., Tyver P.: Acute lithium induced tremor. *Br J Psychiatry*
    143:40–41, 1983.
Vestergaard P.: Clinically important side effects of long-term lithium
    treatment: A review. *Acta Psychiatr Scand (Suppl)* 305:1–36, 1983.

WEIGHT GAIN

Incidence and Presentation

The incidence of self-reported weight gain in the 1st
month of lithium therapy is 30%; in the 5th month, 42%.

The incidence of weight gain in patients on long-term

lithium therapy has been reported to be from 10 to 42%. However, it has been suggested that weight gain tends to occur in patients who experienced weight problems prior to lithium therapy. In one study, 20% of patients receiving lithium gained more than 10 kg body weight during an average period of 5.2 years (Vestergaard et al, 1980).

Mechanism

The exact mechanism is unknown. Proposed mechanisms are:

1. Increased caloric intake secondary to either CNS effects of lithium or stabilization in the patient's psychiatric condition.
2. Increased thirst and polydipsia.
3. Altered carbohydrate metabolism as a result of the insulinlike effect of lithium.
4. Concurrent administration of neuroleptic or anti-depressant medications.
5. Lithium-induced hypothyroidism.

Clinical Significance

Weight gain often results in poor lithium compliance; subsequently, the rate of relapse often increases.

Recommendations

Strict control of diet by limiting caloric intake can result in substantial weight loss. The patients should be under close medical supervision to ensure that they are on an electrolyte-balanced diet, particularly normal sodium intake.

Suggested Readings

Awad A. G.: Diet and drug interactions in the treatment of mental illness: A review. Can J Psychiatry 29:609–613, 1984.

Dempsey G. M., Dunner D. L., Fieve R. R., et al: Treatment of excessive weight gain in patients taking lithium. Am J Psychiatry 133:1082–1084, 1976.

Duncavage M. B., Nasr S. R., Altman E. G.: Subjective side effects of lithium carbonate: A longitudinal study. *J Clin Psychopharmacol* 3:100, 1983.

Vendsborg P. B., Prytz S.: Glucose tolerance and serum lipids in man after long-term lithium administration. *Acta Psychiatr Scand* 53:64–69, 1976.

Vendsborg P. B., Bach-Morteroseo N., Rafaelson O. J.: Fat-cell number and weight gain in lithium treatment patients. *Acta Psychiatr Scand* 53:255–359, 1976.

Vestergaard P., Amdisen A., Schou M.: Clinically significant side effects of lithium treatment: A survey of 237 patients in long-term treatment. *Acta Psychiatr Scand* 62:193–200, 1980.

WITHDRAWAL EFFECTS

Presentation

In one study of symptoms of withdrawal from lithium, 19% of 27 patients who withdrew reported heightened anxiety, irritability, and emotional lability (Christodoulou and Lykouras, 1982). These symptoms suggest a true withdrawal reaction. There is also another report suggesting that lithium withdrawal can trigger psychotic states in patients who have mood swings and minor affective disturbances during lithium therapy (Klein *et al*, 1981). However, there are also studies of abrupt lithium discontinuation in which no withdrawal symptoms were found.

Incidence

The incidence of a true withdrawal syndrome is not known, and the existence of such a syndrome is still controversial. In the aforementioned study of withdrawal symptoms, 19% of patients reported withdrawal-like symptoms when they defaulted from their lithium trial.

Mechanism

The mechanism for withdrawal effects is not known. The effect could be due to a rebound from long-standing biochemical changes caused by the lithium, or a psychological effect in patients who have become emotionally dependent on the drug, or a combination of both. If a true withdrawal syndrome exists, it must arise from a central effect of lithium on the nervous system, with the sudden removal of lithium causing a state of heightened arousal.

Clinical Significance

At present, there is little evidence for a true withdrawal syndrome; nevertheless, there are a few reports suggesting that some patients may experience one. Most patients do not have withdrawal symptoms when lithium is discontinued, and several well-controlled studies do not support the existence of a withdrawal syndrome. More important, when one withdraws lithium from a previously controlled patient, one must be vigilant for signs of relapse in the affective disorder for which lithium was originally prescribed.

Recommendations

Although true withdrawal symptoms are probably infrequent, it might be wise to gradually taper lithium to avoid the possibility of increased anxiety or other rebound phenomenon, particularly if the patient has received lithium for a substantial period of time.

Suggested Readings

Christodoulou G. N., Lykouras E. P.: Abrupt lithium discontinuation in manic–depressive patients. *Acta Psychiatr Scand* 64:310–314, 1982.
King J. R., Hullin R. P.: Withdrawal symptoms from lithium: Four case reports and questionnaire study. *Br J Psychiatry* 143:30–35, 1983.
Klein H., Broucek B., Greil W.: Lithium withdrawal triggers psychotic states. *Br J Psychiatry* 139:255–264, 1981.

MISCELLANEOUS EFFECTS

Alopecia: There is a case report of a 56-year-old female who developed hair loss from various parts of the body despite normal thyroid function. In addition, after 2 months, she noticed the appearance of a rash on her skin. Dermatology treated the condition with topical treatment. Despite continuation of lithium therapy, the hair and skin disorders disappeared.

Ghadiran A. M., Lalinec-Michaud M.: Report of a patient with lithium related alopecia and psoriasis. *J Clin Psychiatry* 47(4):212, 1986.

Anemia: A 40-year-old male patient, maintained on 600–700 mg/day with a lithium level of 1.17 meq/liter, developed megaloblastic anemia that was treated with 15 mg/day of oral folate.

Prakash R., Sethi H., Agrawal S. S., et al: A case report of megaloblastic anemia secondary to lithium. *Am J Psychiatry* 138(6):849, 1981.

Choreoathetosis: Choreoathetosis (irregular jerks or writing movements) has rarely been reported with lithium; it may be more often associated with lithium toxicity.

Zorumski C., Bakris G.: Choreoathetosis associated with lithium: Case report and literature review. *Am J Psychiatry* 140:1622–1622, 1983.

Folic acid deficiency: A letter to the editor questioned the sometimes quoted statement that folic acid deficiency is a side effect of lithium, arguing that no cause-and-effect relationship has been as yet established.

Jefferson J. W.: Is folate deficiency a side effect of lithium therapy? (letter). *J Clin Psychiatry* 47:276, 1986.

Hyperparathyroidism: Several case reports have suggested that lithium is associated with development of primary hyperparathyroidism.

Rothman M.: Acute hyperparathyroidism in a patient after initiation of lithium therapy. *Am J Psychiatry* 139:362–363, 1982.

Sexual dysfunction: Two cases of male sexual dysfunction were characterized by loss of libido and impairment of erection. In the first case, a 42-year-old male was on lithium with levels between 0.7 and 0.9 meq/liter for approximately 16 months before experiencing sexual dysfunction, which remitted with medication discontinuation. In the second case, a 56-year-old bipolar patient was on lithium with serum levels of 0.5 meq/liter for approximately 7 months. After 2 months of continued lithium treatment, symptoms abated.

Sergio B. L., Marcos F. P. T., Calil H. M.: Lithium-induced male sexual impairment: Two case reports. *J Clin Psychiatry* 43:497–498, 1982.

Sialorrhea (Increased salivation): A 37-year-old male with a serum lithium level of 0.85 meq/liter developed a painless swelling of the submaxillary glands and increased salivation with no other side effects. Lithium was discontinued for a month, with salivation returning to normal. Lithium was restarted with hypersalivation, which was treated with propantheline bromide, 15 mg BID.

Donaldson S. R.: Sialorrhea as a side-effect of lithium: A case report. *Am J Psychiatry* 139:1350–1351, 1982.

Thyrotoxicosis: There is a case report of a 57-year-old female who at first developed hypothyroidism after taking lithium for 8 years, then suddenly became thyrotoxic.

McDermott M., Burman K., Hofeldt F., *et al:* Lithium-associated thyrotoxicosis. *Am J Med* 80:1245–1248, 1986.

5

Reactions to Benzodiazepines

BEHAVIORAL EFFECTS

Hostility

Presentation

The emergence of hostile reactions may involve increased verbal hostility and even physical assault. Often this behavior appears to be triggered by some frustrating stimulus before the patient "lashes out." Some patients describe being very restless and pace the room before losing control.

Incidence

The incidence of emergent hostility with benzodiazepines is not known and may depend on the patient's diagnosis, level of frustration, and impulsiveness. In one study, 8 of 80 patients treated with alprazolam became hostile early in their treatment (Rosenbaum *et al*, 1984); most of these patients had a history of chronic anger and suppressed resentment. There are fewer reports of hostility with oxazepam, but this lesser occurrence may reflect the lower potency of this drug, rather than its ability to trigger hostile behavioral reactions.

Mechanisms

Although some of the reports of hostility with ben-zodiazepines may involve drug toxicity, the mechanism appears to involve the disinhibition of behavior and subsequent release of underlying anger and hostility.

Clinical Significance

On the basis of cases reported in the literature, the emergence of hostility with benzodiazepines is not common, but when it occurs, the result may be dramatic. Perhaps more often, the increase in hostility may be slight rather than overt, so that it may be mistaken as a symptom of a psychiatric disorder or even interpreted as an improvement in assertive behavior. For whatever reasons, hostile reactions from benzodiazepines appear more likely to occur in patients with poor impulse control.

Recommendations

Benzodiazepines are useful drugs for treating anxious patients and even those with high levels of aggression. Paradoxically, however, they may trigger unwanted hostility in susceptible patients. The clinician should be aware of this potential, which can occur with all marketed ben-zodiazepines, and consider the possibility of drug-induced hostility when dramatic behavioral reactions are reported in patients taking benzodiazepines. Although controversial, ox-azepam may be less likely to trigger paradoxical reactions. Should such reactions occur, the clinician should also consid-er the possibility of drug intoxication (benzodiazepines and other drugs such as alcohol). Rebound anxiety can also occur when benzodiazepines are stopped abruptly.

Suggested Readings

Goldney, R. D.: Paradoxical reaction to a new minor tranquilizer. *Med J Aust* 1:139–140, 1977.

Lion J. R.: Benzodiazepines in the treatment of aggressive patients. *J Clin Psychiatry* 40:70–71, 1979.

Rosenbaum J. F., Woods S. W., Groves J. E.: Emergence of hostility during alprazolam treatment. *Am J Psychiatry* 141:792–793, 1984.

Sedation

Presentation

Sedation appears to be the opposite of alertness, but it is not an easy concept to define precisely. In addition to an increase in so-called "sleepy" behaviors (e.g., rubbing the eyes, yawning), there is a reduced level of consciousness and impairment of motor coordination, memory, and recall.

Incidence

All benzodiazepines have the potential to cause sedation when given in usual therapeutic doses. Individual sensitivity as well as environmental circumstances may influence the expression of subjective drowsiness or sleepiness. Daytime sedation occurs more commonly when these drugs are taken during the day or when benzodiazepine hypnotics with long half-lives are used the night before.

Mechanism

Sedation appears to result from excessive central nervous system (CNS) depression, probably mediated by interaction with γ-aminobutyric acid (GABA) receptors or the glycine receptor or both. Unlike barbiturates, however, benzodiazepines possess anxiolytic action that is distinct from purely sedative effects alone.

Clinical Significance

Daytime sedation should be avoided in patients who work with heavy machinery or those who must perform fine motor tasks. Patients who drive automobiles may be at risk for increased accidents.

Recommendation

Treatment with benzodiazepines should be tailored to the needs of the individual patient. Dosage should be increased gradually to avoid unnecessary sedation, which poses a risk for increased accidents. In patients treated for anxiety, dosage should be titrated so that the anxiety is diminished without excessive drowsiness. When these drugs are used as hypnotics, the possibility of sedation the following day must also be considered. In this case, benzodiazepines with shorter half-lives cause less daytime sleepiness than those with longer half-lives. With a short-half-life drug, the patient's alertness may even increase during the daytime because, in addition to there being no persisting drug effects, the patient is able to get a good night's sleep. The clinician should also consider whether the patient might be a good candidate for a non-benzodiazepine such as buspirone.

Suggested Readings

Bliwise D., Seidel W., Karacan I., *et al:* Daytime sleepiness as a criterion in hypnotic medication trials: Comparison of triazolam and flurazepam. *Sleep* 6:156–163, 1983.

Greenblatt D. J., Shader R. I., Abernethy D. R.: Current status of benzodiazepines (second of two parts). *N Engl J Med* 300:410–416, 1983.

CARDIOVASCULAR EFFECTS

Presentation

A decrease in systolic blood pressure of 20 mm Hg and decreases in diastolic blood pressure of 3–5 mm Hg have been reported.

Increases in heart rate ranging from means of +3 to +15 beats/min have been reported.

It has been suggested that diazepam given intravenously can dilate coronary blood vessels and enhance coronary blood flow (Ikram, 1973).

When diazepam was given intravenously with comparable doses for anesthesia, an increase in the heart rate and a decrease in blood pressure, stroke volume, left ventricular stroke work, and cardiac output are reported in patients with normal pulmonary function. A decrease in total peripheral resistance was also observed. In patients with obstructive lung disease, left ventricular stroke work, stroke volume, and systolic blood pressure were markedly reduced, but heart rate, diastolic blood pressure, or total peripheral resistance were not reduced (Rao, 1973).

Incidence

Hypotension: The percentage of the total number of patients reported ranged from 0.1 to 4.7%.

Tachycardia and palpitation: The percentage of the total number of patients reported ranged from 0.2 to 7.7%.

Occasionally, transient episodes of bradycardia are reported after rapid intravenous injection of a benzodiazepine, i.e., diazepam (Valium®). A review of the literature indicates that the incidence of changes in heart rate associated with injectable diazepam is relatively rare, i.e., less than 0.2% (Keim and Sigg, 1973).

Mechanism

It is believed that the effects of benzodiazepines on the cardiovascular system, such as resting tachycardia, are mediated primarily through the CNS, rather than through the direct effects on the peripheral autonomic nervous system.

The beneficial effects of benzodiazepines on coronary blood vessels and on myocardial blood flow when given intravenously are mediated locally rather than centrally. The effects of benzodiazepines when given orally to provide symptomatic relief for patients with angina pectoris are probably due to central antianxiety effects instead of a direct effect on myocardial blood flow.

The decrease in left ventricular stroke work, stroke volume, and cardiac output might be due to direct depressive effects of benzodiazepines on the myocardium. The decrease in blood pressure might be due to a decrease in cardiac output.

Clinical Significance

Since few or no significant adverse hemodynamic changes and changes in baroreceptor sensitivity are reported, particularly when care is taken to follow the recommended doses and procedures for administration of benzodiazepines, these drugs are considered to be relatively safe for the cardiovascular system.

Recommendations

Although it is considered that benzodiazepines are less likely to produce cardiovascular depression than barbiturates and the effects are considered to be benign when doses within the recommended range are given orally, physicians administering these drugs must familiarize themselves with the significant hemodynamic changes that can occur in some patients. An individual assessment of cardiovascular function must be performed before prescribing these medications, and when given intravenously, rates of infusion should follow manufacturer's guidelines.

Suggested Readings

Cote P., Gueret P., Bourassa M. G.: Systemic and coronary hemodynamic effects of diazepam in patients with normal and diseased coronary arteries. *Circulation* 50:1210–1216, 1974.

Elliott H. W., Nomof N., Navarro G., Ruelius H. W., Knowles J. A., Comer W. H.: Central nervous system and cardiovascular effects of lorazepam in man. *Clin Pharmacol Ther* 12:468–481, 1971.

Greenblatt D. J., Shader R. I.: Benzodiazepines (first of two parts). *N Engl J Med* 291(19):1011–1015, 1974.

Ikram H., Rubin A. P., Jewkes R. F.: Effect of diazepam on myocardial blood flow of patients with and without coronary artery disease. *Br Heart J* 35:626–630, 1973.

Keim K. L., Sigg E. B.: Vagally mediated cardiac reflexes and their modulation by diazepam and pentobarbital. *Neuropharmacology* 10:319–321, 1973.

Markiewicz W., Hunt S., Harrison D. C., Alderman E. L.: Circulatory effects of diazepam in heart disease. *J Clin Pharmacol* 16:637–644, 1976.

Rao S., Sherbaniuk R. W., Prassad K., Lee S. J. K., Sproule B. J.: Cardiopulmonary effects of diazepam. *Clin Pharmacol Ther* 14:185–189, 1973.

Valium: A monograph. Roche Laboratories, Nutley, New Jersey, 1980.
Wagner B. C., McIntosh H. D.: The use of drugs in achieving successful
    DC cardioversion. *Prog Cardiovasc Dis* 11:431–442, 1969.

RESPIRATORY EFFECTS

Presentation

When sufficient doses of benzodiazepines are given intravenously for anesthesia, respiratory depression can occur, including depression of alveolar ventilation associated with an increase in the arterial carbon dioxide tension and a decrease in pH.

Incidence

The incidence of respiratory depression with injectable diazepam is 0.3%; that of apnea (cessation of breathing) is also 0.3%.

Mechanism

The effects of benzodiazepines on the respiratory system are believed to be mediated primarily through the CNS.

Clinical Significance

When benzodiazepines are administered in the recommended doses, they usually produce no clinically significant changes in respiratory rate or blood gases. With the administration of higher doses, respiratory depression has been reported. Benzodiazepines can enhance depression from narcotics, anesthetic agents, or a narcotic analgesic that is a known respiratory depressant.

Recommendations

When benzodiazepines are administered in higher dosage than recommended to patients who are taking CNS-depressant drugs or who are elderly, seriously ill, or with limited pulmonary function, they can cause significant respiratory side effects, including the possibility of apnea or cardiac arrest or both. Therefore, an individualized assessment must be performed before prescribing the drug. Also, recommended procedures must be followed carefully. Start patients on a low dose, slowly increase the dosage, and prescribe the lowest possible dosage for the maximum therapeutic effect; if the medication is given intravenously, administer slowly over 5–10 min.

Suggested Readings

Clergue F., Desmonts J. M., Duvaldestin P., Delavault E., Saumon G.: Depression of respiratory drive by diazepam as premedication. *Br J Anaesthesia* 53:1059–1063, 1981.

Greenblatt D. J., Shader R. I.: Benzodiazepines (first of two parts). *N Engl J Med* 291:1011–1015, 1974.

Markiewicz, W., Hunt S., Harrison D. C., Alderman E. L.: Circulatory effects of diazepam in heart disease. *J Clin Pharmacol* 16:637–644, 1976.

McClish A.: Diazepam as an intravenous agent for general anesthesia. *Can Anaesthesiol Soc J* 13:562–575, 1966.

Paulson B. A., Becher L. D., Way W. L.: The effects of intravenous lorazepam alone and with meperidine on ventilation in man. *Acta Anaesthesiol Scand* 27:400–402, 1983.

Rao, S., Sherbaniuk R. W., Prssad K., Lee S. J. K., Sproule B. J. L.: Cardiopulmonary effects of diazepam. *Clin Pharmacol Ther* 14:182–189, 1973.

Valium: A monograph. Roche Laboratories, Nutley, New Jersey, 1980.

TERATOGENIC EFFECTS

Presentation

There have not yet been any congenital defects reported with the use of lorazepam, oxazepam, temazepam, lorazepate, or clonazepam.

Chlordiazepoxide: There are reports of spastic diplagia, microcephaly, duodenal atresia, and Meckel's diverticulum.

Diazepam: There are reports of cleft lip/palate, inguinal hernia, cardiac and circulatory defects, hemangiomas, pyloric stenosis, case reports of absence of both thumbs, spina bifida, absence of left forearm, and syndactyly.

Neonatal withdrawal: Withdrawal from the benzodiazepine may occur but is not a teratogenic effect. Due to the slow neonatal metabolism of the drug, the symptoms may not be apparent until a few weeks of age. Symptoms include severe tremulousness, irritability, intrauterine growth retardation, hypertonia, diarrhea, vomiting, and vigorous sucking.

Floppy infant syndrome: Symptoms include hypotonia, lethargy, sucking difficulties, feeble cry, hypothermia, poor reflexes, and apnea.

Incidence

Existing studies are conflicting, suggesting both teratogenicity and absence of teratogenicity. There are no consistent results on which to base a definite conclusion.

Mechanism

These drugs may alter the development of the CNS during organogenesis, during early differentiation, or during biochemical differentation of the brain. The insult to the CNS is commonly thought to be at the time of neural tube closure (during the formation of the primary shape of the CNS).

Benzodiazepines appear to cross the placenta readily.

Clinical Significance

Studies have associated diazepam with cleft lip/palate with drug use during the first and second trimesters. However, other studies have not found this association.

Animal studies revealed that experimental methodology employed had considerable effect on results. One consistent feature in many studies was the need for extremely high doses (from 8 to 300 mg/kg as a single dose or as repeated doses) to produce a teratogenic effect.

It is suggested that exposure to benzodiazepines at any

time during pregnancy may result in visible deformations as well as functional and behavioral deficits.

Recommendation

Benzodiazepine use in pregnancy is controversial, and recent data indicate that its risk to cleft lip may be slight or not related to the drug at all. All benzodiazepines should be used with care in the pregnant patient.

Suggested Readings

Weber L. W. D.: Benzodiazepines in pregnancy—Academic debate or teratogenic risk? *Biol Res Pregnancy Perinatol* 6(4):151–167, 1985.

Briggs G. G., Bodendorfer T. W., Freeman R. K.: in *Drugs in Pregnancy and Lactation*. Baltimore, Williams & Wilkins, 1983.

Onnis A., Grella P.: in *The Biochemical Effects of Drugs in Pregnancy*, Vol I. Ellis Horwood, 1984.

Rosenberg L.: Lack of relation of oral clefts to diazepam use during pregnancy. *N Eng J Med* 309:1282, 1983.

WITHDRAWAL AND TOLERANCE EFFECTS

Presentation

Common withdrawal symptoms noted in the literature include insomnia, agitation, anxiety, tremors, dysphoric mood states, gastrointestinal distress, and perceptual hypersentivities (hyperacusis, photophobia, paresthesias, and hypersensitivities to touch). In addition, severe reactions such as seizures, coma, and psychotic states have been noted with medications such as oxazepam, lorazapam, and triazolam (short plasma half-lives). Symptoms usually emerge within 48 hr after abrupt discontinuation and last for less than seven days; with medications that remain in the body longer (e.g., diazepam, chlordiazepoxide), symptoms may emerge within 2–3 days but may continue for 2–4 weeks. Recognizing withdrawal symptoms can be difficult because the central features of anxiety and insomnia often resemble the condition for which benzodiazepines are prescribed. For example, benzodiazepines (particularly those with short half-lives) used for sleep may cause a rebound insomnia indistinguishable from the original sleep problem. In addition, the patient may claim the drug is no longer effective or that he needs to increase the dosage for the desired effect, which may imply that a tolerance is probably occurring.

Incidence

The incidence of tolerance is not well known, but it appears to be related to the dosage and length of treatment. The incidence of withdrawal symptoms is better documented; they have occurred in 15–44% of patients, depending on the design of the particular study.

Mechanism

There are both psychological and physical mechanisms associated with the development of tolerance and withdrawal from benzodiazepines (sometimes referred to as minor tranquilizers). By definition, tolerance occurs when the dosage must be increased to obtain the same anxiolytic or sedative effect. The withdrawal effect may occur on discontinuation or a rapid decrease in medication. The mechanism for tolerance and withdrawal is incompletely understood, but it appears that withdrawal involves changes in the sensitivity of the receptors and tolerance may be associated with changes in the receptor and increased metabolism with chronic use.

Clinical Significance

Clinicians should be aware of the propensity of these drugs to produce tolerance, which leads to (1) continued use of the drug but without therapeutic effect or benefit, (2) increasing the dosage to obtain the same effect, and (3) the likelihood of withdrawal reactions when benzodiazepines are abruptly discontinued. In general, the incidence of symptoms appears to be low, although addiction-vulnerable patients are at higher risk, especially if they use alcohol regularly or are taking other sedative or pain-relief medications. Tolerance is probably infrequent when treatment is limited to brief periods of time. If a patient has been taking benzodiazepines for three months or more, however, he may be at risk for development of tolerance and subsequent withdrawal reaction. Alprazolam (Xanax) may be associated with a more severe withdrawal reaction than other benzodiazepines, so it is particularly important to taper this drug slowly, particularly when higher dosages are used.

Recommendations

If a patient is at risk for developing withdrawal symptoms because of dosage or length of therapy, it is best to carefully taper the drug slowly (usually decrease the dosage by 25–50% every 3–4 days and monitor for emergence of withdrawal symptoms). Fortunately, most reactions are mild and can be managed by supportive treatment. Severe reactions, however, can be life-threatening, and this condition requires careful medical detoxification. If a short-acting benzodiazepine is involved, it is best to substitute with an equivalent dosage of a long-acting benzodiazepine and then withdraw slowly (see Table 1).

Tolerance can be prevented by careful use of benzodiazepines, limiting the length of treatment and availability of automatic refills. Clinicians can minimize the consequences of developing tolerance to benzodiazepines by monitoring carefully both dosage and length of treatment and by avoiding prescribing these drugs for patients who have a history of substance abuse.

Table 1. Approximate Equivalent Doses[a]

Benzodiazepines	Dose (mg)
Oxazepam (Serax)	15
Chlordiazepoxide (Librium)	10
Diazepam (Valium)	5
Lorazepam (Ativan)	1
Chlorazepate (Tranxene)	7.5
Alprazolam (Xanax)	0.25

[a]Based on comparison of manufacturer's recommended adult dose.

Suggested Readings

Csernansky J. G., Hollister L. E.: Withdrawal reaction following therapeutic doses of benzodiazepines. *Hosp Formulary* 18:900–902, 1983.

Dietch J.: The nature and extent of benzodiazepine abuse: An overview of recent literature. *Hosp Community Psychiatry* 34:1139–1145, 1983.

Dominguez R. O., Goldstein B. J.: 25 years of benzodiazepine experience: Clinical commentary on use, abuse, and withdrawal. *Hosp Formulary* 20:1000–1014, 1985.

Harrison, M.: Diazepam tapering in detoxification for high-dose benzodiapezine abuse. *Clin Pharmacol Ther* 36:527–533, 1984.

Kales A., Scharf M. B., Kales J. D., *et al:* Rebound insomnia: A potential hazard following withdrawal of certain benzodiazepines. *J Am Med Assoc* 241:1692–1695, 1979.

Lader M., Higgitt A.: Management of withdrawal from benzodiazepines. *Int Drug Ther Newsl* 21(6):21–24, 1986.

Noyes R., Perry P. J., Crowe R. R., *et al:* Seizures following the withdrawal of alprazolam. *J Nerv Ment Dis* 174:50–52, 1986.

Rickels K., Case W. G., Downing R. W.: Issues in long-term treatment with diazepam. *Psychopharmacol Bull* 18:38–41, 1982.

MISCELLANEOUS EFFECTS

Amnesia: Six patients were given placebo and six were given 2 mg/day of lorazepam. The lorazepam group recalled fewer words than placebo, supporting the claim that lorazepam may effect short-term recall of verbal material.

Mac D. S., Kumar R., Goodwin D. W.: Anteriograde amnesia with oral lorazepam. *J Clin Psychiatry* 46:137–138, 1985.

Ejaculatory inhibition: In a case report of a 47-yr-old male, when the dose of alprazolam was increased to 1.5 mg TID, the patient reported an inability to ejaculate. The possible mechanisms for this reaction are discussed.

Munjack D. J., Crocker B.: Alprazolam-induced ejaculatory inhibition (letter). *J Clin Psychopharmacol* 6(1):57–58, 1986.

In addition, alprazolam has been implicated in inhibited female orgasm. *Am J Psychiatry* 142:1223–1224, 1985.

Excitatory state: Three patients received 1–3 mg/day of alprazolam and developed an excitatory state within days of initiating therapy. In only one case was there an underlying affective illness. The literature suggests a disinhibition syndrome with benzodiazepines. However, in these cases, symptoms suggestive of mania are apparent. The authors suggest a neurochemical link between mania and disinhibitory states.

Straham A., Rosenthal J., Kaswar M., *et al:* Three case reports of acute paroxysmal excitement associated with alprazolam treatment. *Am J Psychiatry* 142:859–861, 1985.

Hostility: Of 80 patients treated with alprazolam, 8 became hostile. The dose ranged from 0.5 to 8 mg/day.

Rosenbaum J. F., Woods S. W., Groves J. E., *et al:* Emergence of hostility during alprazolam treatment. *Am J Psychiatry* 141:792–793, 1984.

Manic episodes: Two bipolar patients developed mania after 20–35 days of treatment with 2.5–4 mg/day of alprazolam.

Arana G. W., Pearlman C., Shader R. J.: Alprazolam-induced mania: Two clinical cases. *Am J Psychiatry* 142:368–369, 1985.

Alprazolam, an antianxiety drug that has been claimed to have antidepressant activity, has been noted to precipitate mania in depressed patients and in patients treated with this drug for agoraphobia and panic disorder.

Pecknold J. C., Fleury D.: Alprazolam-induced manic episode in two patients with panic disorder. *Am J Psychiatry* 143:652–653, 1986.

Stuttering: The patient was taking alprazolam 0.25 mg BID and 0.5 mg at bedtime for 4 days, experienced increased anxiety, and took an additional 1 mg alprazolam and began to stutter. The stuttering stopped 2 days after the medication was discontinued for 2 days.

Elliot R. L., Thomas B. J.: A case report of alprazolam-induced stuttering. *J Clin Psychopharmacol* 5(3):159–160, 1985.

6

Reactions to Antiparkinson Agents

AUTONOMIC EFFECTS

Cardiovascular Effects

Presentation and Mechanism

The cardiovascular effects are dose-related. Low doses can cause transient bradycardia; moderate or high doses can cause tachycardia, palpitation, and arrhythmias (due to blockage of vagal effects on the S-A node).

Serious antiparkinson agent overdoses are often associated with electrocardiographic (ECG) abnormalities, including widening of the QRS complex, prolonged QT interval, and ST segment depression.

Clinical Significance and Recommendations

Older patients who have a compromised cholinergic function, or patients who already have diseases of the cardiovascular system, are more prone to the development of cardiac side effects with antiparkinson agents. Therefore, for sensitive patients, low doses of antiparkinson agents should be administered initially and doses then titrated gradually. Also, monitor ECG changes and cardiac status closely.

Gastrointestinal Effects

Presentation and Mechanism

The gastrointestinal (GI) effects are dose-related. These effects include dryness of the mouth, nausea, vomiting, difficulty in swallowing, hiatal hernia (due to the anticholinergic activity at the esophagus and gastric sphincter), constipation, fecal impaction, and paralytic ileus (due to the reduction of motility and tone of the GI tract as well as the volume of its various secretions).

Clinical Significance and Recommendations

Avoid prescribing antiparkinson agents for elderly patients or patients with debilitated physical condition, megacolon complicated by ulcerative colitis, obstructive diseases of the GI tract such as pyloric stenosis, and hiatal hernia with reflux esophagitis.

Ocular Effects

Presentation and Mechanism

The ocular effects are dose-related and include cycloplegia, i.e., paralysis of accommodation (due to the paralysis of the ciliary muscles of the lens), mydriasis, photophobia, blurring of vision (due to the effects on the eye involving responses of the radial fibers and the sphincter muscle of the iris), and an increase in intraocular pressure. The latter may precipitate or aggravate a crisis in patients with narrow-angle glaucoma (due to the blockage of the drainage of aqueous humor through the angle of the anterior chamber of the eye).

Clinical Significance and Recommendations

The severity of the narrow-angle glaucoma crisis depends on the degree of anticholinergic effect on the pupils and the dose of the drug.

Avoid prescribing antiparkinson agents for patients with narrow angle glaucoma. Patients with open-angle glaucoma (which is independent of the size of the pupils) usually tolerate antiparkinson agents without significant adverse effects, particularly when the glaucoma is adequately treated. If administration of antiparkinson agents to patients with narrow-angle glaucoma that has been properly treated is absolutely necessary, intraocular pressure must be monitored closely.

Dermatological Effects

Presentation

These agents can cause cutaneous vasodilation, particularly at toxic doses (known as "atropine flush"). It is not known whether this vasodilation is a response to help dissipate an increase in body temperature or whether it is a direct effect on cutaneous vessels. There is also an inhibition of sweat gland secretion, resulting in reduced volume of perspiration. At toxic doses, there may be suppression of sweating, resulting in an increase in body temperature.

Recommendations

1. Avoid high doses of combined antipsychotics and anticholinergics, particularly during hot summers.
2. Certain environments with high humidity cause more of a problem because of a decreased ability to evaporate sweat.

Urological Effects

Antimuscarinics decrease the tone and amplitude of contractions of the ureter and bladder, commonly exhibited as complaints of urinary retention. (These agents also inhibit penile erection and may produce impotence.)

Recommendation

A decrease in dosage may help ameliorate the severity of this effect.

Suggested Readings

Hall R. C. W., Feinsilver D. L., Holt R. E.: Anticholinergic psychosis: Differential diagnosis and management. *Psychosomatics* 22:581–587, 1981.

Hiatt R. L., Fuller I. B., Smith L., *et al:* Systemically administered anticholinergic drugs and intraocular pressure. *Arch Ophthalmol* 84:735–740, 1970.

Lamy P. P.: Update on antiparkinsonian agents. *Geriatr Pharmacol* 37:81–91, 1982.

Shimomura S. K., Siepler J. K.: Parasympatholytic cholinergic blocking agents in Knoben J. E., Anderson P. O. (eds): *Handbook of Clinical Drug Data,* 5th ed. Hamilton, Illinois, Drug Intelligence Publications, 1983, pp 376–378.

Van der Kolk B. A., Shader R. I., Greenblatt D. J.: Autonomic effects of psychotropic drugs, in Lipton M. A., DiMascio A., Killam K. F. (eds): *Psychopharmacology: A Generation of Progress,* 2nd ed. New York, Raven Press, 1978, pp 1009–1020.

Weiner N.: Atropine, scopolamine, and related antimuscarine drugs, in Gilman A. G., Goodman L. S., Rall T. W., Murad F. (eds): *The Pharmacological Basis of Therapeutics,* 7th ed. New York, Macmillan, 1985, pp 130–144.

Zaratzian V. L.: Drug-induced dysfunctions of the autonomic nervous system, in Blum K., Manzo L. (eds): *Neurotoxicology.* New York, Marcel Dekker, 1985, pp 69–81.

EUPHORIC EFFECTS

Presentation

Patients who were prescribed antiparkinson agents for extrapyramidal side effects refused discontinuation of the drugs because of lethargy or depression or because they "did not feel as well" without the drugs. They reported a dose-related energizing state that alleviated a depressed state. One patient reported a "high" experience that induced an animated and pleasantly hallucinogenic state (Jellinek, 1977, 1981).

Incidence

The incidence of euphoric effects is unknown. There have been several case reports describing mood-altering effects.

Mechanism

The mechanism of these effects is unclear. It has been suggested that cholinergic pathways related to the regulation of affect in the central nervous system play a role in altering affective states.

Clinical Significance and Recommendations

Clinicians should evaluate each patient who is on neuroleptics for the presence of extrapyramidal effects and the need for anticholinergic medication. Avoid prescribing anticholinergic agents routinely for all patients taking neuroleptics. Be aware of the abuse potential of antiparkinson agents, particularly with patients who have a past history of substance abuse.

Evaluate the need for prolonged maintenance on antiparkinson agents periodically.

When discontinuing an antiparkinson agent, the drug should be decreased gradually to prevent symptoms of withdrawal from the drug as well as a dysphoric state (akinetic depression) resulting from the recurrence of extrapyramidal side effects.

Suggested Readings

Goggin D. A., Solomon G. F.: Trihexyphenidyl abuse for euphorigenic effect. *Am J Psychiatry* 136:459–460, 1979.

Jellinek T.: Mood elevating effect of trihexyphenidyl and biperiden in individuals taking antipsychotic medication. *Dis Nerv Syst* 38:353–355, 1977.

Jellinek T., Gardos G., Cole J. O.: Adverse effects of antiparkinson drug withdrawal. *Am J Psychiatry* 138:1567–1571, 1981.

MacVicar K.: Abuse of antiparkinsonian drugs by psychiatric patients. *Am J Psychiatry* 134:809–811, 1977.

Rubinstein J. S.: Abuse of antiparkinson drugs. *J Am Med Assoc* 239:2365–2366, 1978.

TERATOGENIC EFFECTS

Incidence

There is no information on incidence due to lack of studies.

Mechanism

The general concern is when these agents are given during the first trimester of pregnancy, which is the period for organogenesis.

Clinical Significance

There are no controlled studies available in humans or animals.

Recommendations

1. Use antiparkinson agents with care during pregnancy, since their safety has not been established.
2. These agents should probably be used only if the potential benefit justifies the potential risk to the fetus.

Suggested Readings

Briggs G. G., Bodendorfer T. W., Freeman R. K., *et al: Drugs in Pregnancy and Lactation: A Reference Guide to Fetal and Neonatal Risk.* Baltimore, Williams & Wilkins, 1983.

Heironen O. P., Slone D., Shapiro S. (eds): *Birth Defects and Drugs in Pregnancy.* Littleton, Massachusetts, Publishing Sciences Group, 1977.

Omnis A., Grella P. (eds): *The Biochemical Effects of Drugs in Pregnancy,* Vol I. New York, John Wiley, 1984.

The Royal Women's Hospital Reference Guide on Drugs in Pregnancy. Carlton, Victoria, R. Batagol, 1983.

MISCELLANEOUS EFFECTS

Mental side effects: A survey of the mental side effects of amantadine in 295 hospital employees found that 30 reported some mental symptoms. The most frequent side effect was elevation of mood in 47% of the 30; there was decrease in mood, increase in energy, or hypersomnia in 41%. Other side effects noted were night terrors and disturbances in memory and orientation, and 7% of the 30 employees experienced delusions.

Flaherty J. A., Bellur S. N.: Mental side effects of amantadine therapy: Its spectrum and characteristics in a normal population. *J Clin Psychiatry* 42(9):344–345, 1981.

Neuroleptic malignant syndrome: A case is reported of neuroleptic malignant syndrome that developed in a 50-year-old male after discontinuation of amantadine and neuroleptic. At the time of discontinuation, the patient was hyperpyrexic with elevated temperature and mental confusion.

Simpson D. M., Davis G. C.: Case report of neuroleptic malignant syndrome associated with withdrawal from amantadine. *Am J Psychiatry* 141:796–797, 1984.

7

Major Psychotropic Drug Interactions

ANTIPSYCHOTICS

Interacting substance(s)	Mechanism	Clinical significance	Recommendation
Alcohol	Additive CNS effect, particularly sedation.	May impair driving performance or other activities that require concentration.	The combination may be used, but continual monitoring is required
Anticoagulant	Enzyme induction with haloperidol and enzyme competition with phenothiazines.	May increase or decrease coagulation effect, depending on antipsychotic used.	Close monitoring of prothrombin time.
Anticonvulsants (Phenobarbital, Phenytoin, Carbamazepine, Mysoline)	Enzyme induction.	May decrease antipsychotic plasma level, which may result in relapse.	Monitor clinical symptoms and plasma levels for antipsychotic and anticonvulsant. Dosage adjustments may be necessary.

(continued)

ANTIPSYCHOTICS *(Continued)*

Interacting substance(s)	Mechanism	Clinical significance	Recommendation
Antihypertensive (Guanethidine)	Prevention of guanethidine reuptake in presynaptic membrane.	Decreased antihypertensive effect.	Monitor blood pressure; switch to another antihypertensive agent.
β-Blocker	Reported with thioridazine and chlorpromazine; possible enzyme competition.	May cause an increase in antipsychotic plasma level.	Precautionary monitoring of antipsychotic side effects.
Disulfiram	Interaction is associated with perphenazine; however, may occur with other phenothiazines. Enzyme inhibition is responsible for this interaction.	May lead to an increased effect of antipsychotic.	Monitor target symptoms and adjust dosage.
L-Dopa	Both drugs affect striatal dopamine receptors and are mutually antagonistic.	May increase psychosis or decrease antiparkinson effects.	Monitor psychosis and parkinsonian symptoms. Consider thioridazine or other low-potency antipsychotic medication.
Epinephrine (IV)	Not a pure α-agonist.	If blood pressure is low, epi-	Avoid IV use of epinephrine.

(continued)

ANTIPSYCHOTICS (Continued)

Interacting substance(s)	Mechanism	Clinical significance	Recommendation
		nephrine may further lower blood pressure.	May be safer to use α.
Tobacco	Enzyme induction.	If the patient decides to stop smoking, there may be an increase in drowsiness, or orthostatic hypotension. In addition, heavy smoking may lead to reduced antipsychotic effect	Monitor side effect and therapeutic effects and adjust dose accordingly.

ANTIDEPRESSANTS
Tricylic and Tetracyclic

Interacting substance(s)	Mechanism	Clinical significance	Recommendation
Alcohol	Additive synergistic effect.	Misinterpretation of target symptoms and side effects.	Caution patient about operating hazardous machinery or driving an automobile.
Antihypertensive (Bethanidine, Clonidine, Guanethidine)	May inhibit the uptake of certain antihypertensives, particularly beth-	Decreased antihypertensive effects.	Switch to another antihypertensive agent.

(continued)

ANTIDEPRESSANTS
Tricylic and Tetracyclic (*Continued*)

Interacting substance(s)	Mechanism	Clinical significance	Recommendation
	anidine and guanethidine.		
Monoamine oxidase inhibitors	1. Enhance effects of tricyclic antidepressant. 2. Tricyclics may sensitize adrenergic receptors to amines.	Symptoms of hyperpyrexia, excitability, muscular rigidity, alteration in blood pressure; in rare instances, may be lethal.	1. Monitor patient closely. 2. Rule out medical risks. 3. Consider the combination only after conventional treatments have failed.
Oral anticoagulant	Inhibition of hepatic microsomal enzymes.	Enhanced effect of oral anticoagulation.	Monitor prothrombin time shortly after initiating therapy and weekly for approximately 1 month.
Sympathomimetic (epinephrine)	Not a pure α-agonist in the sympathetic nervous system.	May further decrease blood pressure.	Avoid IV use of epinephrine.
Tobacco	Enzyme induction.	See **Antipsychotics.**	See **Antipsychotics.**

ANTIDEPRESSANTS
Monoamine Oxidase Inhibitors

Interacting substance(s)	Mechanism	Clinical significance	Recommendation
Alcohol	Additive CNS depression; increase in tyramine with certain wines and beer.	May lead to over-sedation or even coma if a large amount is ingested; may lead to hypertensive crisis with certain alcoholic beverages.	Avoid significant alcohol consumption. Avoid consuming Chianti red wine, sherry, and certain beers and ales with high tyramine content.
L-Dopa	Increased storage and release of catecholamines.	May lead to hypertensive crisis (see *Tyramine* below).	Always use carbidopa with L-dopa to inhibit peripheral decarboxylation.
Meperidine or dextromethorphan	Unknown; may involve increased brain serotonin or increased brain levels of free narcotic.	May lead to development of encephalopathy, convulsions, coma, and respiratory depression.	Avoid the combination.
Sympathomimetics (e.g., epinephrine, norepinephrine, phenylephrine)	Increased storage and release of catecholamines.	May lead to hypertensive crisis (see *Tyramine* below).	Avoid the combination; caution the patient that many OTC drugs contain sympathomimetics; monitor blood pressure.

(*continued*)

ANTIDEPRESSANTS
Monoamine Oxidase Inhibitors (Continued)

Interacting substance(s)	Mechanism	Clinical significance	Recommendation
Tyramine-containing foods	Increased storage and release of catecholamines.	Hypertensive crisis may result (throbbing headache, severe hypertension, tachycardia, sweating, hyperpyrexia; possible rupture of intracranial vessels and death).	Avoid the combination. Instruct the patient to avoid tyramine-rich foods such as aged cheeses, caviar, herring, and sausages, certain alcoholic beverages, fava beans, and certain yeast extracts such as marmite.

LITHIUM

Interacting substance	Mechanism	Clinical significance	Recommendation
Alcohol	Enhanced CNS depression.	May lead to problems in motor coordination or traffic accidents.	Avoid significant alcohol intake when receiving lithium salts.
Antipsychotic	Unknown.	There are several reports of neurotoxicity with haloperidol and thioridazine; however, careful surveys	The combination of lithium and a neuroleptic should be used whenever the patient requires such

(*continued*)

LITHIUM (Continued)

Interacting substance(s)	Mechanism	Clinical significance	Recommendation
		have failed to confirm the significance of this interaction for the major-ity of patients.	treatment, but it would be wise to avoid high doses of antipsychotics and to monitor for develop-ment of neu-rotoxicity.
Carbamazepine	Increased carba-mazepine tox-icity; mechanism unknown.	A few case re-ports describe patients who develop confu-sion, disorien-tation, and diplopia (dou-ble vision).	This combina-tion may have a beneficial therapeutic ef-fect (syner-gism) in some patients; how-ever, it would be wise to monitor blood level of both drugs as well as to assess clinical signs.
Methyldopa	Unknown; idio-syncratic tox-icity with no increase in blood levels.	Increased risk of lithium tox-icity.	Monitor lithium levels to avoid toxicity.
Nonsteroidal antiinflam-matory agents (e.g., indo-methacin, phenylbutazone, piroxicam)	Reduced renal lithium clear-ance.	Studies indicate that lithium levels may in-crease by 30–60% when anti-inflam-matory drugs are added; li-	Monitor lithium levels; it may be necessary to lower the dosage of lithium when adding anti-inflammatory

(continued)

LITHIUM (Continued)

Interacting substance(s)	Mechanism	Clinical significance	Recommendation
		thium toxicity may result.	drugs.
Thiazide diuretic	Reduced renal lithium clearance.	Lithium levels may increase within several days after diuretics are added.	Monitor lithium levels. Lithium patients needing antihypertensives should probably be given a β-blocker, instead of thiazides.
Xanthine (aminophylline, caffeine, theophylline)	Enhanced renal excretion of lithium.	Lithium levels may be decreased by xanthines, leading to decreased antimanic effect.	Monitor lithium levels.

BENZODIAZEPINES

Interacting substance	Mechanism	Clinical significance	Recommendation
Alcohol	Additive CNS depression.	Increased drowsiness, incoordination, risk for accidents.	Avoid alcohol consumption, especially when driving.
Cimetidine	Decreased metabolism of benzodiazepines that are metabolized	Increased benzodiazepine effect, possibly leading to drowsiness,	Use benzodiazepines that are eliminated by phase II type reactions

(continued)

BENZODIAZEPINES (Continued)

Interacting substance(s)	Mechanism	Clinical significance	Recommendation
	by phase I reactions.	incoordination, and other effects.	(e.g., not metabolized by the liver), such as lorazepam and oxazepam.
Digoxin	Decreased metabolism and elimination of digoxin.	Increased plasma levels of digoxin, resulting in enhanced digoxin effect.	Monitor plasma levels of digoxin.
Disulfiram	Decreased metabolism of benzodiazepines that are metabolized by phase I reactions.	May lead to increased benzodiazepine effect.	Use oxazepam or lorazepam to avoid enhanced benzodiazepine effect.

SUGGESTED READINGS

Dukes M. N. G. (ed): *Meyler's Side Effects of Drugs,* 10th ed. New York, Elsevier, 1984.

Evaluation of Drug Interactions, 2nd ed. Washington, DC, American Pharmaceutical Association, 1976.

Jefferson J. W., Greist J. H., Baudhuin M.: Lithium interactions with other drugs. *J Clin Psychopharmacol* 1:124–134, 1981.

Knoben E., Anderson P. O. (eds): *Handbook of Clinical Drug Data,* 5th ed. Hamilton, Illinois, Drug Intelligence Publications, 1983.

Rizack M. A., Hillman C. D. M. (eds): *The Medical Letter Handbook of Drug Interactions.* New York, The Medical Letter, 1983.

Index